T0159484

indulgent

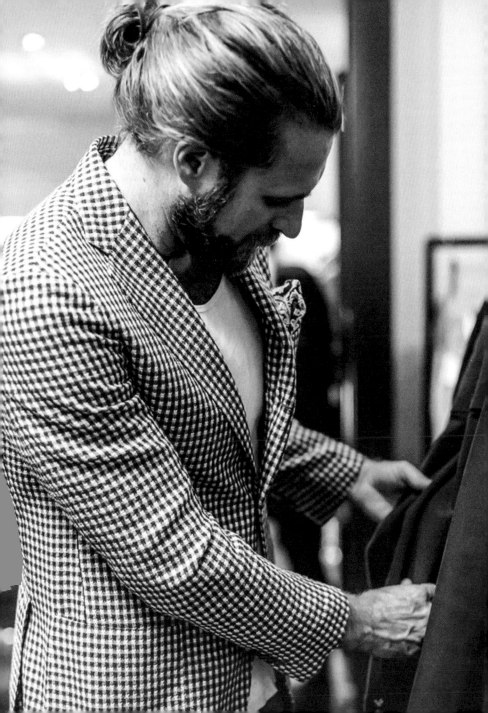

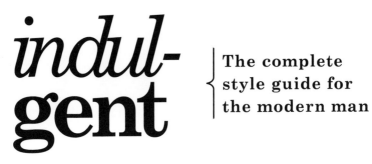

indul-gent

The complete
style guide for
the modern man

JEFF LACK

Contents

Contents

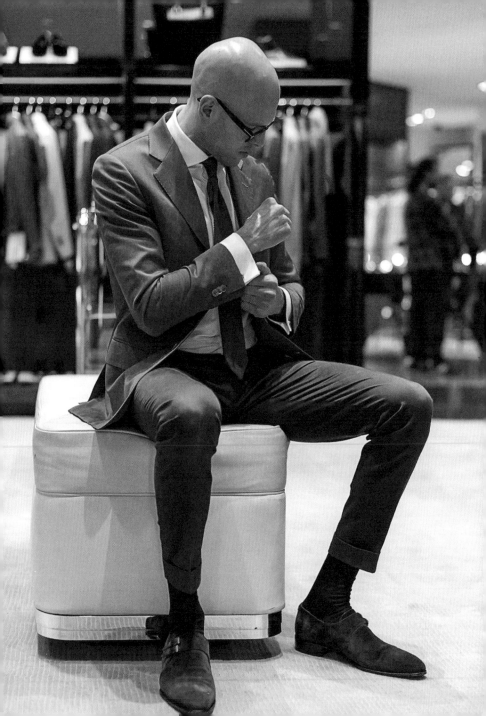

FOREWORD

What does it mean to be a man in the 21st century? Is it about what you do for a living, is it the car you drive, your conquests, your physique, where you live? Yes, some may see these as benchmarks of the modern man—but perhaps there is another way to look at this, which does not include how much coin is in your wallet or how much you can bench-press at the gym.

In the past a gentleman would be expected to express his personality through his sense of style. There was a social expectation and a conscious decision to always put your best foot forward—literally.

The term 'Sunday Best' came from getting dressed up in your best outfit to go to church. This was an opportunity to pull out your sharpest threads and dress to impress. This was often followed by a social meeting where men would gather and chat about current affairs and the week that had been.

There was pride in the appearance of a gentleman that was about the effort they made to look their best.

When did it become ok to 'not care'? The 1960s and 70s, the era of the alternative lifestyle and rejection of the conventional, introduced a different way of thinking about appearance. Comfort over appearance became the trend. Nowadays, it's pretty much anything goes. The 'metrosexual' movement in the early 90s shone light on the subject of style and personal grooming for men.

The effort you make really does go a long way. Often a lot further than you think. Grooming, hair and the overall ensemble for dressing can and does represent how we perceive ourselves as men.

Men today are taking more care of themselves and their appearance proud of what they wear and who they are. When we value ourselves, others can value us too.

So, I'm inviting you to aspire to be your personal best. Your personal style is a billboard for who you are.

This book is a style guide for men of every race and background, white collar, blue collar, no collar! The *indulgent* reader is interested in his appearance. He is every man who wishes to develop his own style.

I hope this book becomes your 'style bible'. Refer to it for fresh ideas for special event styling, shopping trips, wardrobe makeovers and styling tips that have proved successful in my role as a professional stylist. I believe the book can help empower men to be better lovers, brothers, fathers and sons.

My career in fashion spans 25 years and for the past 10, I have worked as a freelance fashion stylist. I wrote this book to share my experiences and my knowledge with you, the reader.

It is the same journey that I take my clients on.

To date I have had the great pleasure in assisting this positive change in my friends and particularly my clients and wish to share as much as possible with you, the reader.

Enjoy
Jeff Lack

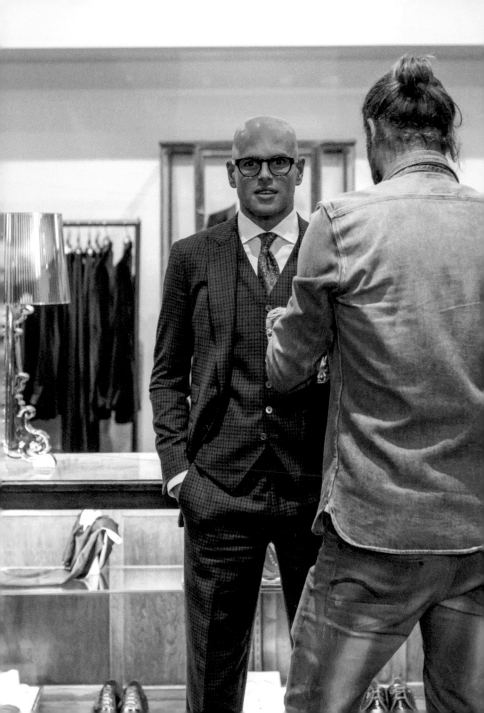

Chapter One

CREDIBILITY

Credibility—this is your personal brand exposed. Credibility connects strongly to first impressions. What is it? How do you show it?

Credibility is about being believed. It's about authenticity, legitimacy and trustworthiness and it comes from being honest with yourself and others. It is the connection between what you do, who you are and how people see you.

If we are talking about personal dress style, credibility is what it means to the real you; to dress in an age-appropriate manner that reflects who you are right now.

Wearing just a little of your personality in your choice of apparel shows the world who you are. How do you see yourself? Are you conventional? Are you an outdoors person? Can your look be conveyed non-verbally through your clothing or accessory choices?

Say for example you're a surfer. You spend every spare moment in the water, but you work in the finance sector.

There is a very definite dress code and standard for this industry: suit and tie. As a self-identified surfer, how could you add a little of this personal side of your life into your business wardrobe. Perhaps you could wear some cool cuff links with something that connects you to your fun-loving surfer side. Don't be afraid to add some spice to your everyday 'work' wardrobe even if your workplace is governed by a fairly regimented dress code.

When people are attracted to another person's energy, it's often largely about how they look. If you are like me, you are interested and drawn to a person because you can feel their confidence and authenticity. That person comes across as credible. There is synergy between their look, and their presentation.

When people meet you, do they 'get' you? Do they see the connection between your personality, how you present, your image and the message you are sending? Do they recognize your credibility and authenticity? Is there a strong correlation between what you say and how you look? When there is a connection, with no distractions, you come across as credible. It's about sending a clear message and being real.

TAKEAWAYS

- Get real, don't kid yourself.
- Create synergy between who you are and how you look.
- Wear your personality on your sleeve.
- Wear age-appropriate clothing.

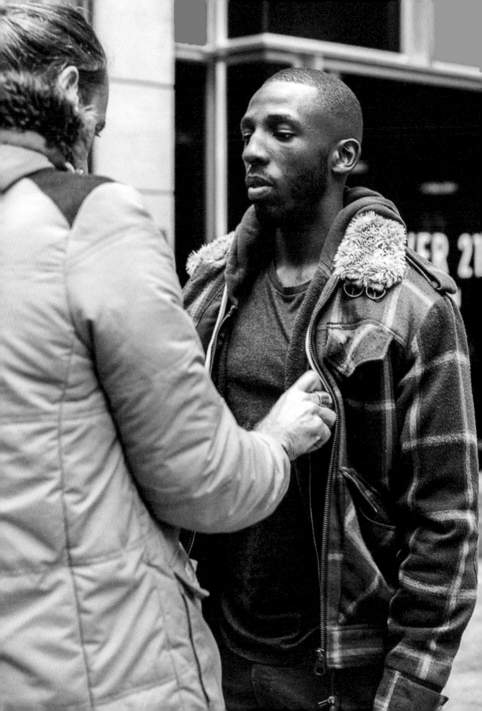

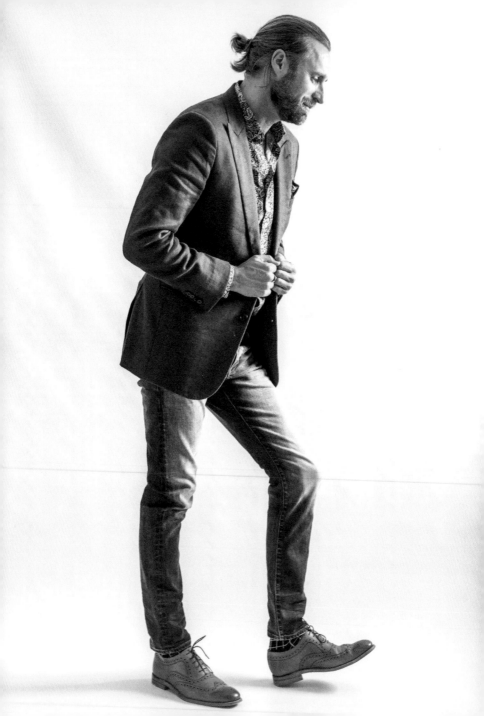

Chapter Two

FIT, COLOR, STYLE

How do you best assess what colors suit you best? How do you understand what is flattering for your body shape? What is your personal style?

I devised the 'fit, color, style' assessment tool in 2007, as I needed to articulate the creative process around individual, unique personal styles. Everyone is different; no two bodies are the same any more than two personalities are the same. We each have a unique code that I believe I can unlock with these tools. I hope this helps you understand how to best represent yourself. When you see someone who looks 'well put together', you can't necessarily put your finger on what it is. That person simply looks good always looking healthy even when they are having a bad day. Such people have the three elements all working: fit, color, style.

FIT

Fit is the most important part of the equation. We can all make an Armani suit look bad if it doesn't fit properly. The fit lines are the key focal points that our eye is drawn to when we look at or meet a person. These are important for aesthetics as well as comfort.

We have all seen trouser hems being eaten up by the pavement because they are too long. We have also seen dudes who can't actually do the top button up on their business shirt because it's too tight. Splitting seams under the pressure of being too tight, or baggy seats of trousers that are too loose—these are the key fit lines that you would do well to have fitting perfectly.

A guide to well-fitted apparel

- *Collars (can fit one finger inside when fastened)*
- *Cuffs (to fit a watch comfortably)*
- *Waist (can fit at least one finger in when fastened)*
- *Seat (just enough room to sit comfortably and not pull)*
- *Hems (no more than one break onto the shoes—too much break means too many folds in the pant leg where it meets the shoe. More than one? Too much break.)*
- *Shoulders (no overhang off the shoulder)*
- *Chest (no pulling or gaping)*
- *Jacket length (finish at your knuckles)*
- *Sleeve length (hits the wrist bone)*
- *Girth (no pulling or straining around the widest part of your belly)*

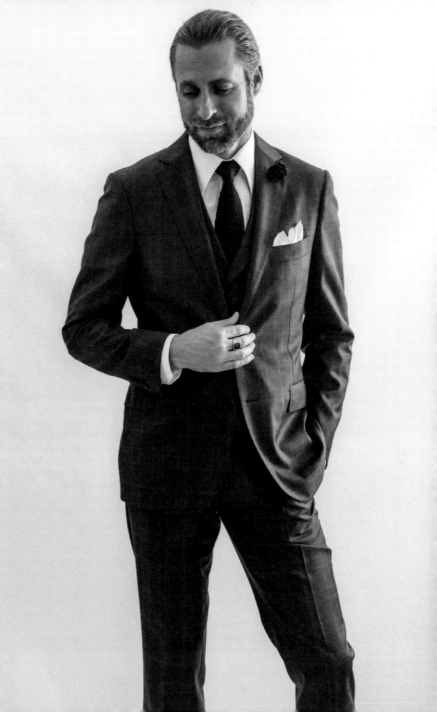

COLOR

Your coloring is the combination of your hair color, eye color and skin tone that creates a base for half a dozen really great colors that you can wear well and that really suits your particular coloring. This is about the colors you wear around your face, as it doesn't matter so much what you wear below.

Beware of colors that are similar to your skin tone as they wash you out. The same applies for really strong contrasts. Look for colors that are soft on your skin; colors that give you a healthy glow. Drape block colors around your neck to see what work best. If you like a color but it drains you, try breaking it up with white or black between the color and your skin.

STYLE

Style is that particular *je ne sais pas*, that something that expresses your personality, your personal image, your personal story. It's about your authenticity, your honesty, a visual connection to your personality. How do you wear your personality literally on your sleeve?

I recommend that you don't let fashion wear you; instead you choose fashion that suits your personal style. The latest fashion won't always suit you. Some fashions are just the wrong cut or color and it's best to sit these out. This is fine as there will be more choice next season. And if you choose some classic pieces, they'll last across many seasons.

When you create the style that is uniquely you, occasional fashion top ups are all you really need to stay inspired, fresh and contemporary.

TAKEAWAYS

■ Assess yourself, no one knows you better than you.

■ Fit is paramount so get it right. Tailoring is key to a perfect fit.

■ Know your coloring and what colors suit you best.

■ Your style is not governed by the latest trends.

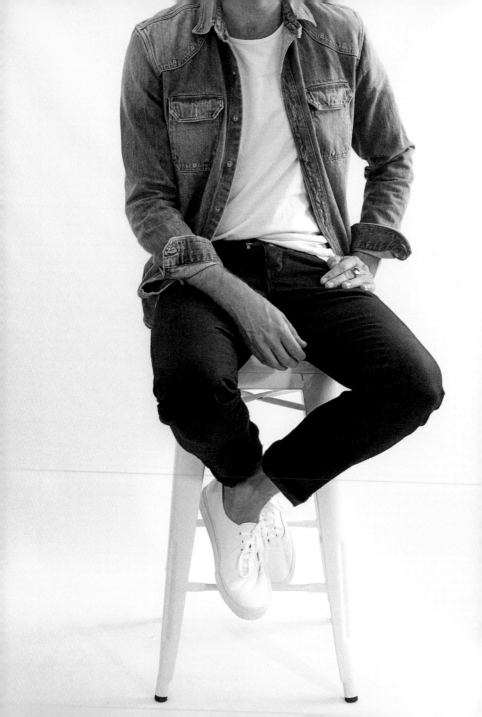

Chapter Three

COLOR ME GOOD

Color can literally change your day! It impacts on you and those you interact with. It can be positive and uplifting when executed well. In the scheme of things, color is the second most important decision when creating an image of your 'best self'. Have you ever worn a shirt that attracts compliments more than anything else in your wardrobe? Consider why. No doubt, it has a lot to do with the color you are wearing.

These days the combination of colors that 'were never to be seen' are *avante guard*. Some examples: black and brown, black and blue, blue and green. These are now worn together and can look sensational.

Beware however of colors that you may love but they may not love you back. Have you ever put a color on that drains you and makes you look a little ill? On another person, it works. On you, it's a no no.

There are some fail-safe 'go-to' color combinations that you can consider if you are unsure. The images in this chapter show you how some color combinations can work well.

Keep an eye on the inspiration hub (chapter 22) with ideas about where to source latest trends and try something different now and then. You never know what killer combination is accidentally (or deliberately) about to transpire.

Try three different shades of blue in good lighting. Perhaps even take a photo of each of them (with your phone, of course) to see which one has the most positive impact on your skin tone. One will certainly look better than the others. Move on to pink and do the same thing. You will see a pattern form as you find whether full rich hues or light pastel hues or something in between will just seem to look better whether it's blues, pinks or greens. In 'wardrobe essentials' you'll see the must-have colors, then all you need to do is apply the above to build a wardrobe of colors that suits you and serves you well.

TAKEAWAYS

■ The colors you wear around your face will impact on how healthy you look.

■ Work with tried and proven color combinations.

■ Try blocks of color around your face to determine what suits you best.

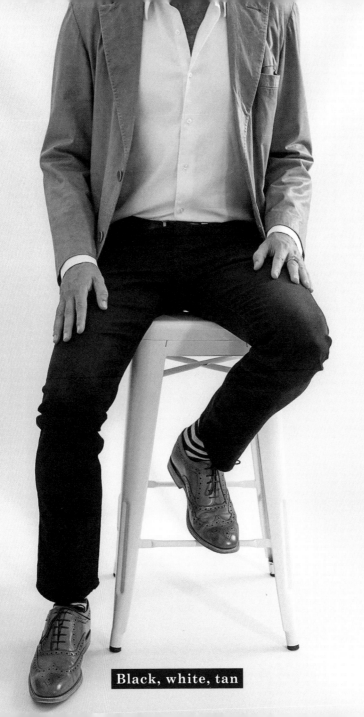

Black, white, tan

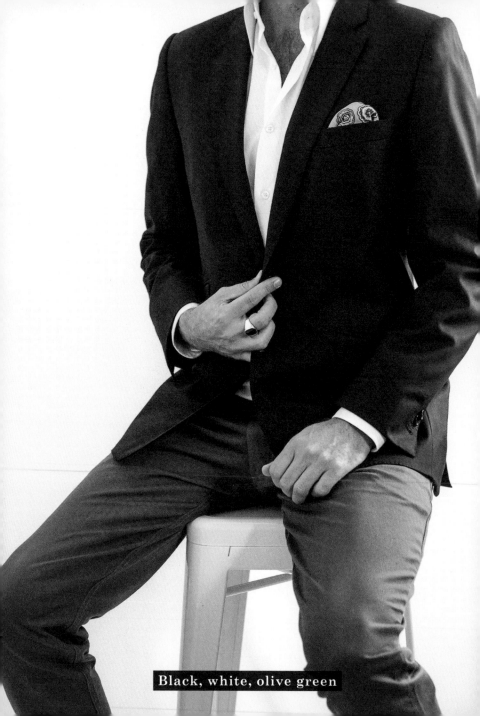

Black, white, olive green

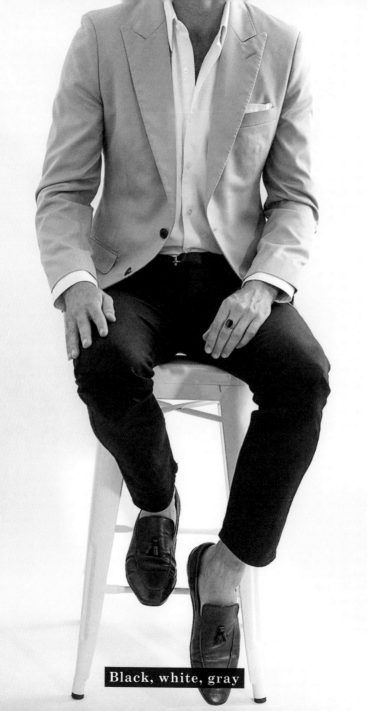

Black, white, gray

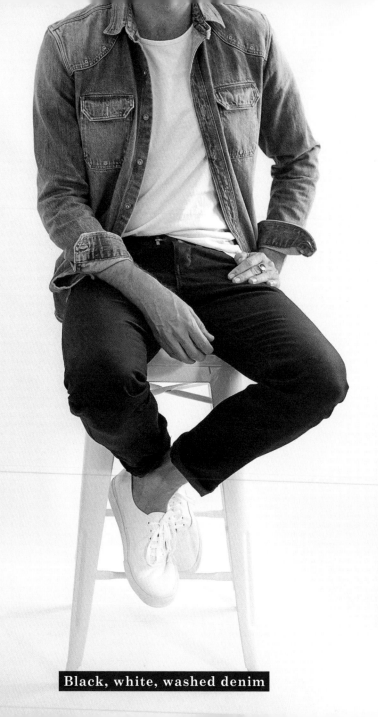

Black, white, washed denim

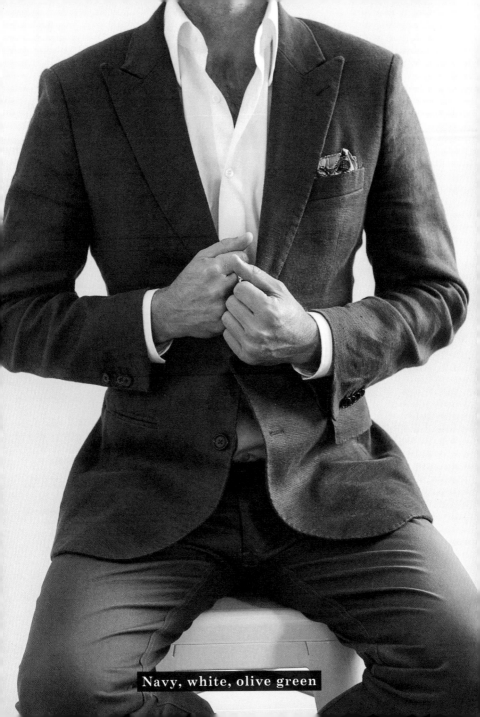

Navy, white, olive green

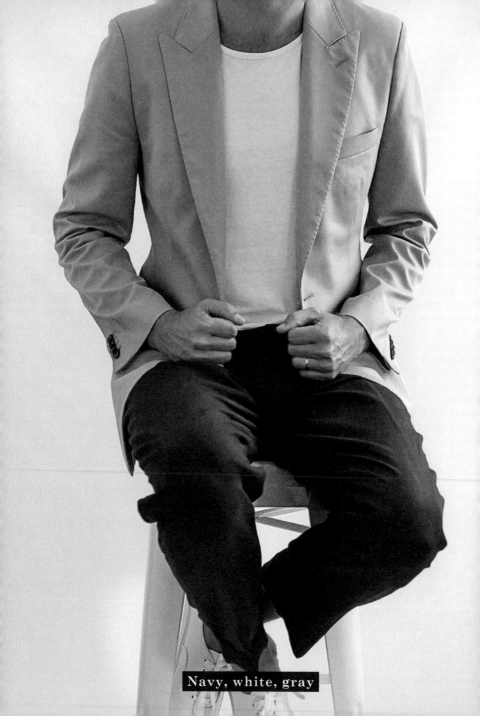

Navy, white, gray

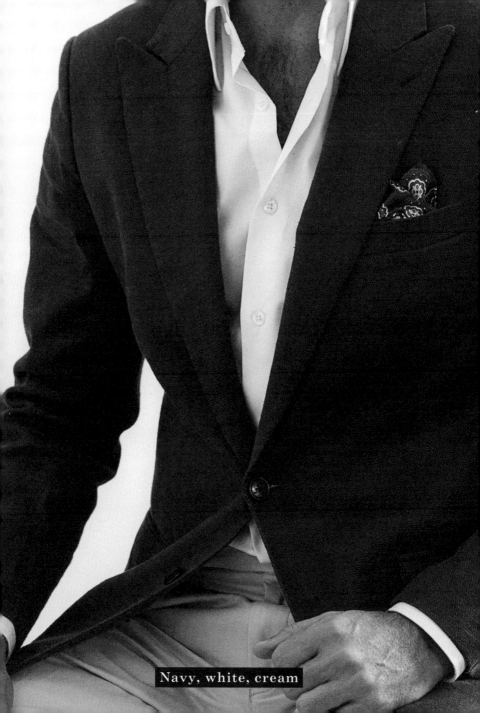

Navy, white, cream

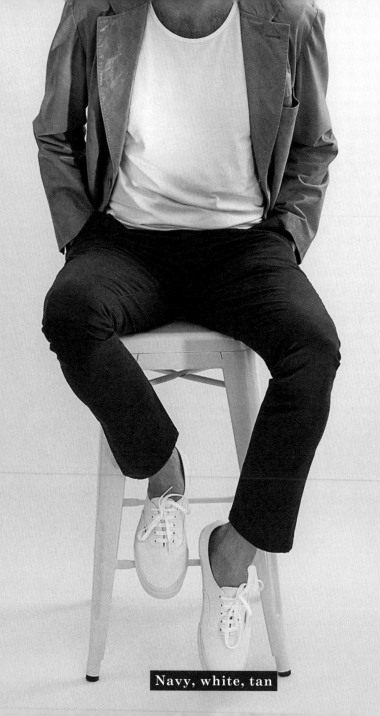

Navy, white, tan

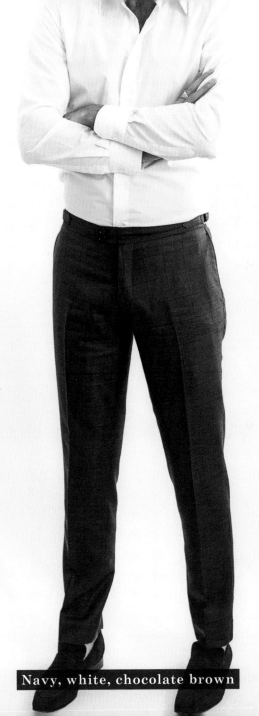

Navy, white, chocolate brown

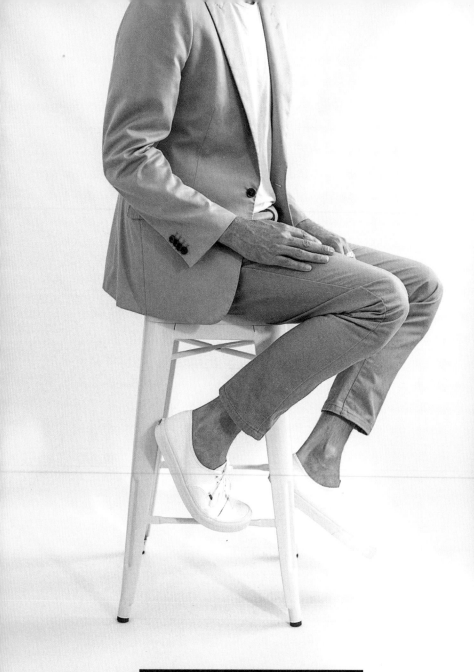

Silver gray, white, lime green

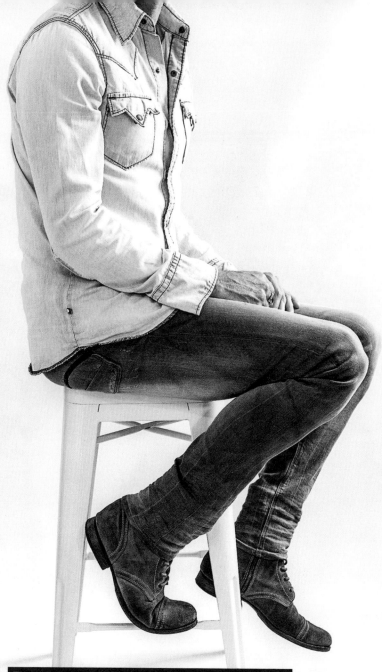

Denim on denim—must be contrasting

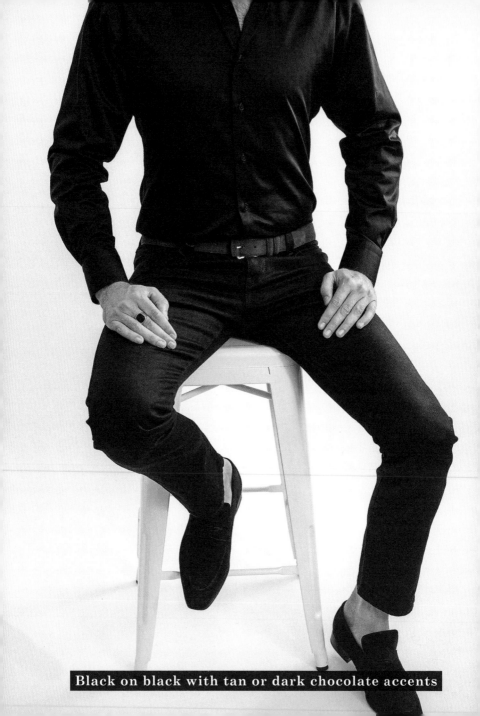

Black on black with tan or dark chocolate accents

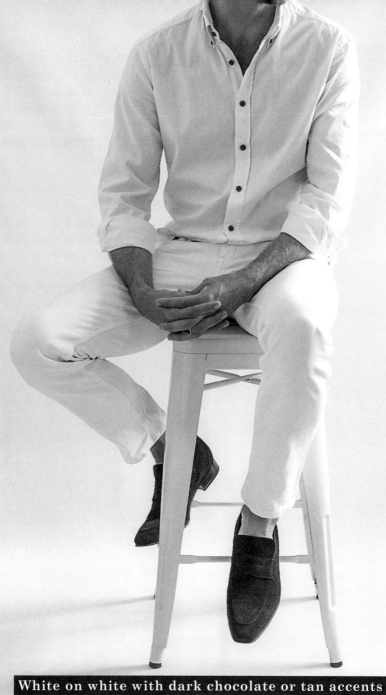

White on white with dark chocolate or tan accents

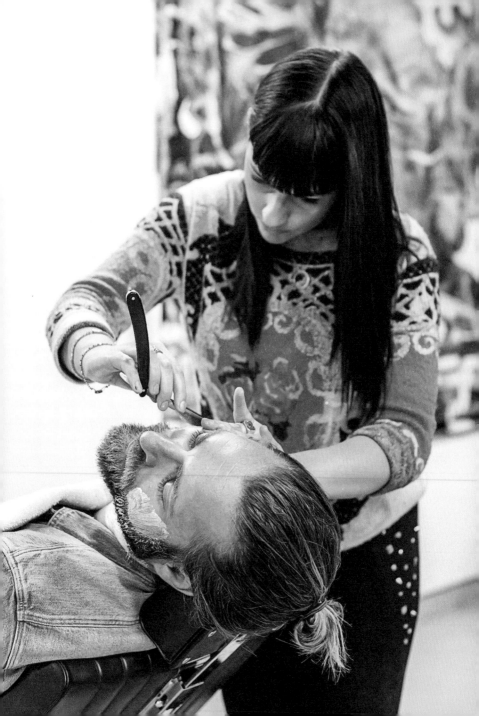

ROUTINE GROOMING

In a world where so much emphasis is put on appearance, it's no longer just the domain of the metrosexual to use hair and skin products—it's now the norm for many men. Moisturizers, eye creams, exfoliating scrubs, night creams, pomade and beard oil are going to keep your skin and hair looking fresh and youthful.

There is no stigma attached to caring about how you look; there's rather an expectation that you do. Besides, a clean shave and some moisturizer can help cloak a hangover.

RECOMMENDED GROOMING ROUTINE

What are the minimum requirements for the modern gent in relation to grooming? What should your grooming routine look like?

Daily

- *Shower every day (body wash rather than soap).*
- *Use underarm deodorant.*
- *Wash your face with cleanser.*
- *Brush and floss your teeth.*
- *Wear sunscreen and/or a moisturizer every day—there are moisturizers that do both. Wash this off in the evening and apply a night cream for face and eyes.*
- *Wear cologne every day as this becomes your signature.*

Weekly

- *Shampoo hair 2–3 times a week (hair usually looks best day three just before you wash it).*
- *Clip facial growth or shave your face 2–3 times per week.*
- *Exfoliate your face 2–3 times a week (exfoliate cream has a grainy texture that removes the top layer of dead skin).*

Fortnightly

- *Clip or cut your fingernails and toenails. Long nails look unattractive and collect dirt more than short nails.*

Monthly

- *Get a haircut or trim and be sure to tend to the eyebrows at the same time.*
- *Have ear and nose hair waxed (I like to say no to Yoda).*
- *Pre-book next month's haircut and hair removal appointment in advance. Behind every decent haircut is a very good hair stylist.*
- *Suffice to say, stay on top of the man jungle downstairs too. A neat trim would suffice.*

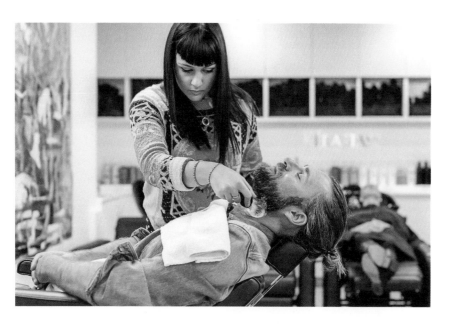

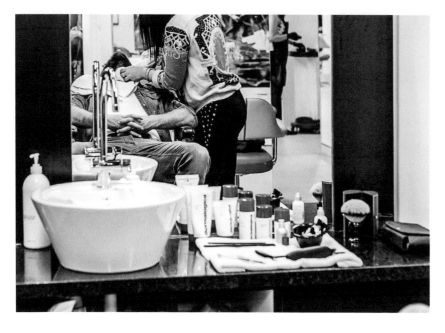

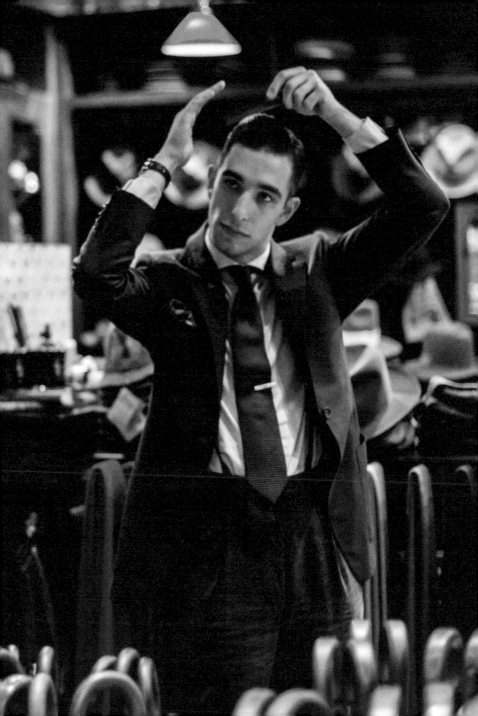

Quarterly

- *Get a new toothbrush. Shaggy, bacteria-filled, worn out toothbrushes tell your visitors that you are unkempt. Keep a bunch of new toothbrushes in your bathroom cabinet.*

Yearly

- *Get a facial on your birthday (this will bring a youthful glow to your skin for a couple of days at least). Have more frequent facials (every three months) if you are so inclined.*
- *Whiten teeth, particularly if you are a red wine or coffee drinker and get a scale and clean with your annual check up at your favorite dentist.*

YOUR HAIR

What about your hair or lack of it when it comes to grooming? What's the modern man's approach?

Styling

For keeping your hair in the shape you desire, try a wax, pomade or clay. Keep in mind that less is more. You can get your hair stylist to show you how much and how to apply when you're next in the salon or barbershop.

Gel is no longer the styling product of choice for the modern man. That haircut that you felt worked for you in 2005 isn't necessarily doing you any favors right now.

Talk to your stylist about getting an inspirational new look or ask about changing your look if you're stuck in a rut.

Balding

Be diligent here, just clip short for a buzz cut on settings #1 or #2 or shave it off completely.

Beards

From a three-day growth to the full beard, beards are the bad boys of fashion. A beard provides a strong masculine look that defines and provides structure to the jaw. For a man with a weak jaw line or double chin, a beard is a godsend.

Whether you choose to go with a beard, or shave your head, you can punch well above your weight when it comes to looking your best.

Many an average-looking dude is doing just that with the combined 'shaved head with beard' look.

HAIR TREATMENTS

What's the latest when it comes to having treatments to protect your hair or replace your hair?

Injectables and fillers

This not a process you want people to recognize straight up. "The idea here," says grooming expert and creative director at Detail for Men, Stephen Foyle, "is to have regular weekly injections so as to not draw attention to the work being done. Subtlety is key.

If people can notice it, we have failed. You can't get away with the three-monthly pumped up no expression fillers and injectables job."

Hair transplants

"Up to 40 percent of clients are thinning or balding," says Foyle. There are real options for balding gents now. Transplants are now done on an individual strand-by-strand basis, grafting from the back of the head which means a much more natural look to the hairline. Topical applications are available that say they can slow hair loss and stimulate the production of hair cells from the root.

Alternatives such as oral applications are reaping better results than ever before. The investment is more affordable than ever and this makes it an actual choice whether you lose your hair or not.

Good grooming isn't about being overly groomed. One should not look too groomed, just well put together. Good consistent grooming is a considered approach with the emphasis on the finer details.

Your grooming regime will pay dividends at work and play, so get started today!

TAKEAWAYS

- With good grooming, you feel and look better.
- Develop a grooming routine.
- Buy quality products, they really do make a difference.
- Your audience will appreciate it.

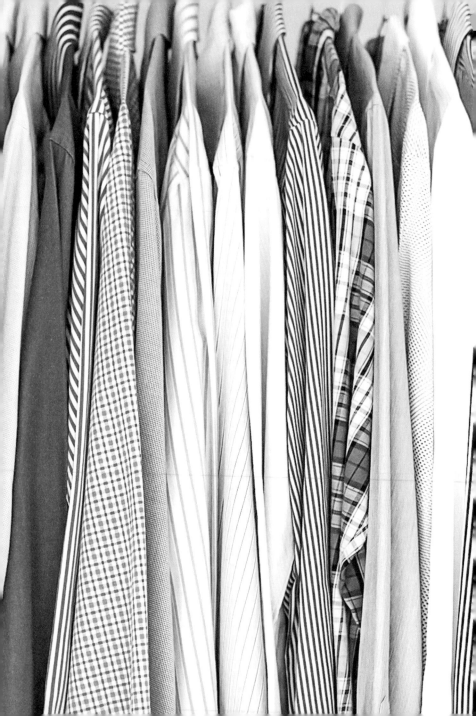

Chapter Five

WARDROBES THAT WORK

"Honey, where are my socks?" We have all struggled from time to time to find pieces in our disorganized wardrobes. So, how do we get our wardrobes to work?

An effective foundation starts with how you organize the actual space in your wardrobe. It should be a reliable utility that reflects you and your personality, so look after this space and your wardrobe will look after you.

If you are working the traditional five days a week, your collection of clothing should represent this. Typically 70 percent will be for work, 30 percent of your collection is for evenings and weekends. Even if you wear smart casual to work, there should be some pieces that you reserve for social occasions. It sometimes helps to keep some space between work and play outfits.

A guide to making your wardrobe work

- *Get the right hangers to suit the space and clothing.*
  Good quality hangers are an important investment.
- *Lay out your wardrobe so you can access every piece*
  without sending out an APB to locate a pair of socks.
  Accessibility is key.
- *At the end of each season, clean out the pieces that no*
  longer serve you each season. These can be re-purposed
  through your charity of choice.
- *Pack up out-of-season goodies so there is more room and*
  access for the current season's collection.

USE A MIRROR EVERY DAY

Ideally your mirror will be in close proximity to your
wardrobe so you can make quick effective changes.

It's incredible how many people walk out the door not
knowing (or just hoping) what the bottom half and back of
the outfit looks like. I see lots of ill-fitting trouser seats,
waistlines, jackets too short and hems and socks that just
scream epic failure!

A full-length mirror will avoid disaster—consider it a
must have in your wardrobe.

A check list before you go out

- *Check your belt is through all the loops.*
- *Check your socks are not tucked into your trouser legs.*
- *Check your shirt is tucked in evenly.*
- *If you're wearing a suit, check that the top and bottom*
  colors match.

COLLECTION OF FLAT LAY SHOOTS

Sometimes we just need a little inspiration and at other times, we need a reminder of what pieces we put together previously for that killer outfit. Creating a collection of flat lay shoots allow you to capture and permanently record complete looks for future reference.

Simply lay the shirt down flat, then butt the trousers up to the shirt, lay the belt and shoes either at the bottom of the trousers (or for a tighter shot next to the waistline). Inside the shoes you can place a pair of socks that match. If there is a jacket to add, lay it down first and place the shirt inside the jacket and add the tie and or scarf as well.

It is best to combine looks, which include shoes, socks, pants, belts, shirts, jackets, scarves and hats. Try as many different combinations as possible and shoot them as a collection for each season.

You will find this system particularly useful when you are packing for a domestic or international flight, as you have outfits that you can match up to the events in your itinerary.

Phones these days have cameras and photo libraries making it easier than ever to record your flat lay shoots.

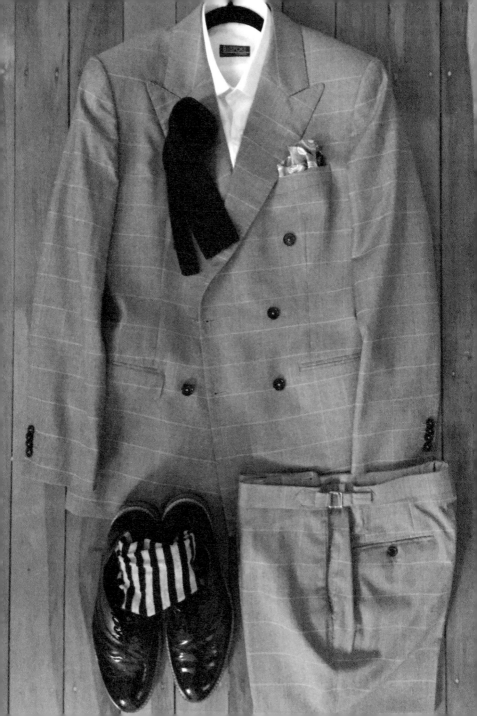

TAKEAWAYS

- Make your wardrobe accessible—create space to move and operate in your wardrobe.

- Your wardrobe should reflect your personality, so look after this space and your wardrobe will look after you.

- Use good quality hangers.

- Pack up and store out of season collections.

- Segment your wardrobe so you can easily find all of your pieces.

- Clean out your wardrobe each season and re-purpose through a charity.

- Photograph your combinations to keep a record of outfits that work.

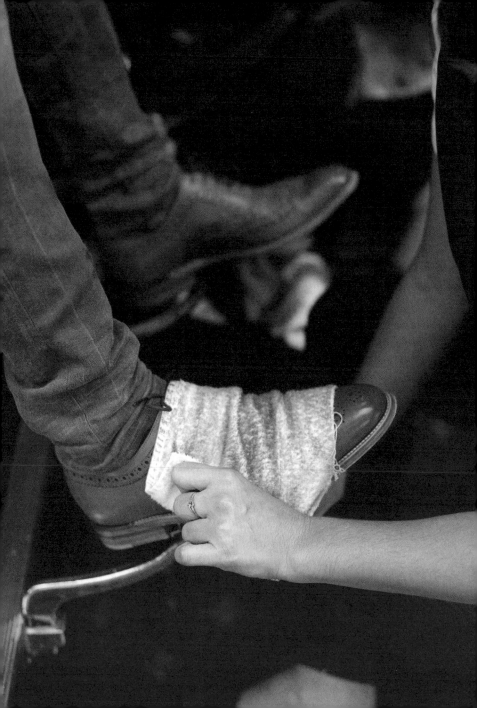

Chapter Six

PROTECT YOUR WARDROBE

How do you look after your wardrobe from footwear, to suits and knitwear? How often should you dry clean your suits? How do you protect your clothing from moths and silverfish? What about washing your favorite jeans? How do you best store clothing?

Continuing the minimalist theme of 'less is more', with fewer good quality pieces in your wardrobe essentials, the easier it is to protect and maintain all your pieces.

Your favorite pair of beat-up jeans are one thing but if you drop $500 on a Gucci shirt, you want to take some care to get the best out of it. High-ticket items like shoes, suits, leather jackets and velvet blazers last longer and feel better with some tender loving care.

We invest in our wardrobes both emotionally and financially. You don't want to be outsmarted by a micro-creature that's just looking for a feed—creepy crawly critters don't discriminate between Lagerfeld and Zara.

When you arrive home from a holiday and find you have lost a bespoke suit to silverfish, or lost shoes to mold, tragedy is not too strong a word to use. However, there are ways to prevent this.

LOOKING AFTER YOUR THINGS

You can be the 'protector' or 'gatekeeper' of your clothing world.

The two main things you can do to protect your wardrobe is to make sure you store your clothing and footwear properly and, when it comes to cleaning, clean apparel carefully so you have the garments you love for a long time to come.

A guide for storing your clothing and shoes

- *Separate your seasons so that there is a little breathing room for your clothing.*
- *Store out-of-season clothing in airtight vacuum bags that will save space and keep your clothing safe.*
- *Hang trousers, shirts, suits and blazers on quality hangers—ideally with a little space between each.*
- *Use shoe trees for good quality hand-made or bespoke footwear. Your shoes will keep their shape longer. Shoe trees can be purchased where you buy your shoes or from a cobbler.*

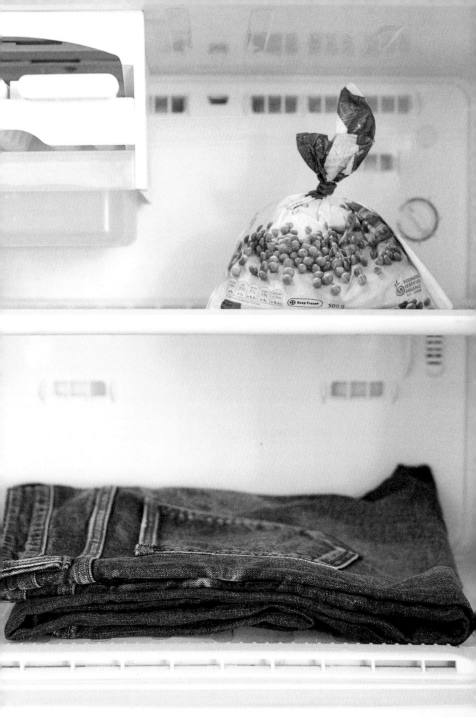

- *For longer wear of your leather-soled shoes, have a half rubber sole fitted a couple of months after you have broken them in. It's important for the leather to scratch up and stretch before you fit the rubber over the top.*
- *Be diligent and change your protection against pesky critters each season. Natural products such as lavender oil or hanging moth balls can help or you may need something more lethal.*
- *High humidity is guaranteed to create mold on clothing and shoes. Mold and mildew love leather so keep an eye on shoes and clean them with a dry cloth. Use a brush for suede. Ventilation is the key to keeping mold to a minimum.*
- *Check the Internet for natural products that can help prevent silverfish or reduce moisture in your wardrobe.*

CLEANING YOUR GARMENTS

When it comes to keeping your garments looking clean and fresh, make sure you check the care instructions on garments and follow them. Front loader washing machines are gentler on your garments and give them longevity.

A guide to washing and drying garments

- *Wash your dark colors and light colors separately.*
- *Use a pre-wash spray for collars, cuffs and stains on shirts or soak overnight for best results. Note that if you spray and immediately wash something, the pre-wash spray does not become active and is rendered useless.*
- *Use eco-friendly washing powder or detergent and cold water.*

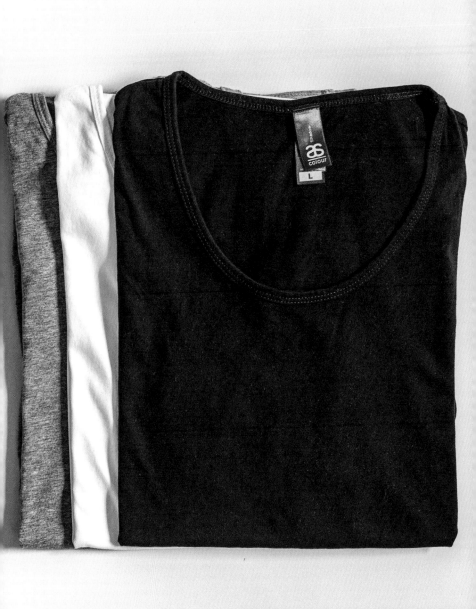

- *Don't leave your clothes to dry in the washing machine as the creasing will be set and difficult to iron, and they can smell damp even after drying.*

- *Dry clean as little as possible as the cleaning fluids and pressing shorten the life of suits in particular. You can ask for 'press only' if the suit is crushed but not too dirty.*

- *Dry garments inside out if you need to dry your clothing in the sun—drying in the shade is best for dark colors.*

- *Dry clean jackets and trousers that are lined as linings and cloth respond differently to water and heat and can shrink leaving the lining showing and/or sagging.*

- *Wash denim sparingly and dry in the shade inside out. Try airing them in between washes on a rack or throw them into a bag in the freezer for a couple of days to help with the odor. Black and raw denim should be left as long as possible without washing because the color comes out every time you wash.*

- *Wash your favorite cotton and woven shirts—anything precious to you—in garment wash bags. Buttons and zips can damage other clothing in the same cycle, so its best to play it safe and separate the delicate pieces.*

- *Hand wash woolens and knitwear in lukewarm water. Do not tumble dry. Lay flat on a drying rack to dry so that it doesn't mark or stretch.*

To wrap up this chapter on maintaining your treasured wardrobe pieces, respect your clothing, treat all your pieces with tender loving care and they will serve you well for many years.

TAKEAWAYS

- Look after your investment if you expect a return on it.
- Don't cut corners: treat your wardrobe with TLC.
- Store your clothing and shoes properly.
- Always read and consider the care instructions on garments and wash and dry them accordingly.

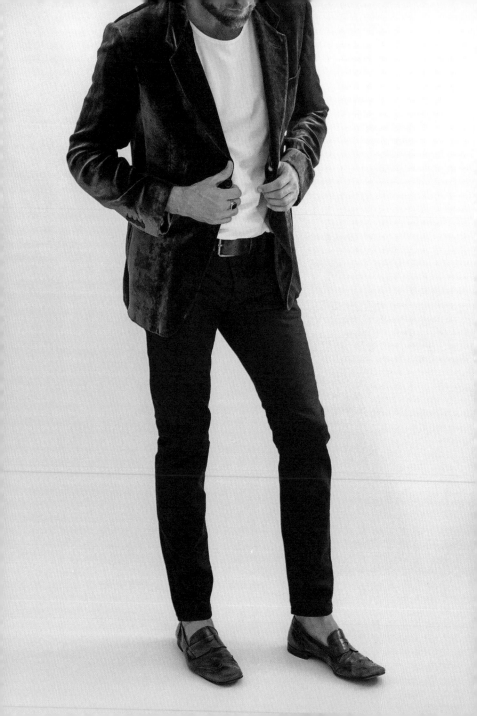

Chapter Seven

32 WARDROBE ESSENTIALS

What are the minimum key pieces for a modern gent's wardrobe? What are the most versatile pieces you need to cut across everyday life and combine to cover multiple events through the seasons?

The mantra for this chapter is 'practical, minimalist, no clutter, fewer choices for more action, confidence and power'.

When making wardrobe decisions, be efficient and you'll be filled with confidence—and compliments will follow.

For your wardrobe, there are some basics that you'll need. Build on these each season and when you need something special for an event, you'll have it covered. When you are building your wardrobe, invest in big-ticket items for suits, coats and footwear. The old adage, "buy once, buy right" means you'll keep your essentials for many years. Also depending on where you live, the weather will prioritize other key pieces.

SUITS

The first three 'must have' suits are: black, navy and mid-gray in plain block colors. The versatility of a single-breasted black suit is the reason you need one. And jackets in block colors will double well as blazers.

I have no problems with business suits being pin striped or checked; it's just when you separate them, the jackets can look badly mismatched.

If your working environment allows for a fashion suit and you have the 'kahunas', go for a colored suit (think cobalt blue or forest green). The combination of these colors will be bold on its own. When split into separates, the jacket would be super cool as a blazer and the trouser could be perfect for a summer cocktail event.

BLACK WOVEN BUTTON-UP LONG SLEEVE SHIRT

A quality black shirt can be worn with suits, jeans or shorts. It makes an ideal sexy evening staple. A nice strong collar is key. Make sure it is not too loose fitting for the smart to formal style. A casual black woven shirt can be a slightly looser fit with a soft collar—try with shorts and chinos. For the adventurous, try pairing your black woven shirt with a black blazer and black jeans for a rock-n-roll vibe.

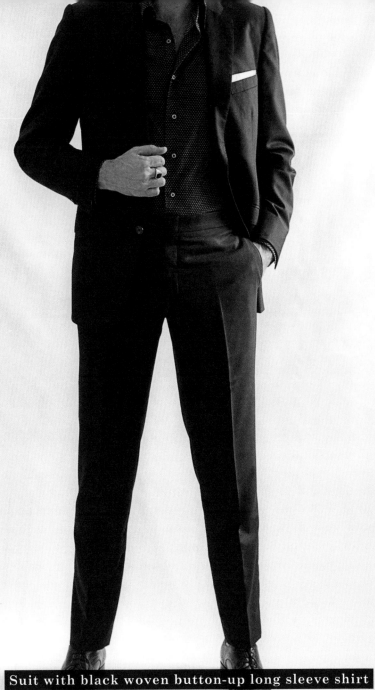

Suit with black woven button-up long sleeve shirt

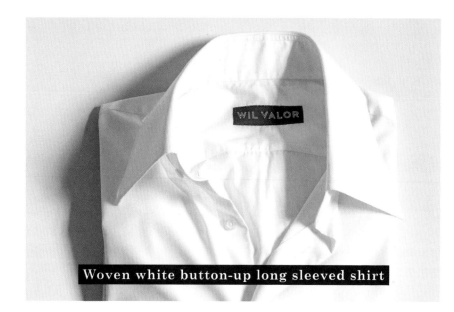

Woven white button-up long sleeved shirt

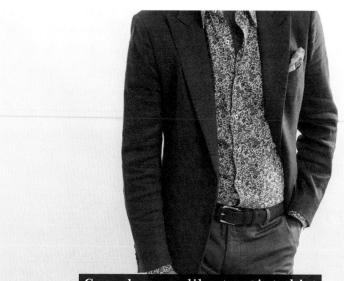

Casual woven liberty print shirt

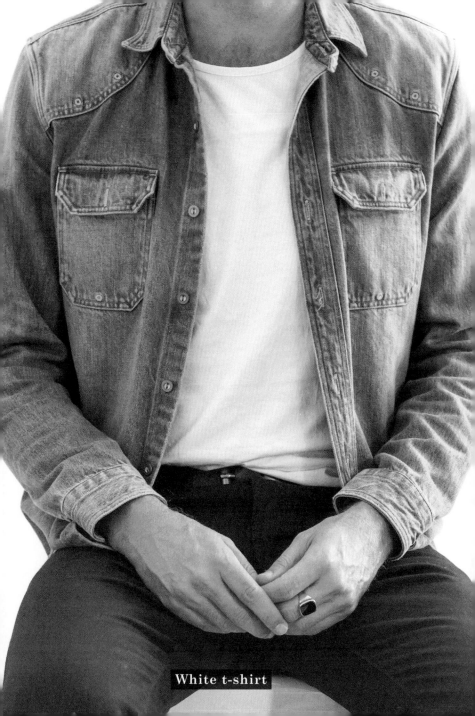

White t-shirt

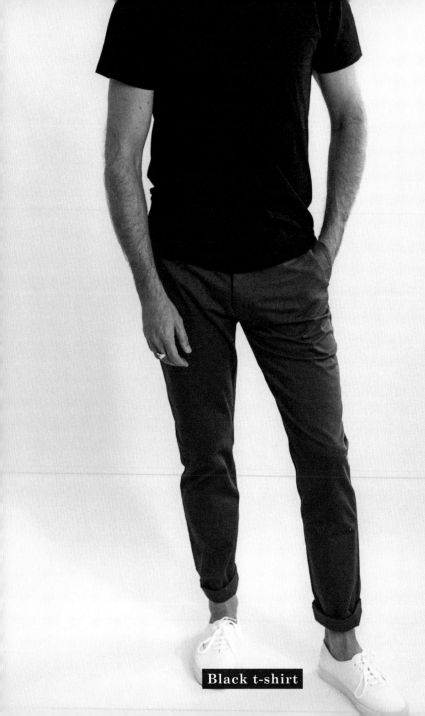

Black t-shirt

WOVEN WHITE BUTTON-UP LONG SLEEVED SHIRT

A white shirt is a must in your wardrobe and should be replaced as the collars and cuffs wear out and or when they take on a yellowish hue.

Make that three white shirts: one formal, one business and one extra casual white shirt.

Wear your white shirts with shorts, jeans, chinos, trousers and suits.

If you are having a shirt made (bespoke) try a contrast button (navy/ charcoal), which will freshen up your denim and chino looks.

CASUAL WOVEN LIBERTY SHIRTS

From swim trunks to chinos to suits, liberty shirts are super versatile. The liberty print woven shirt is not typically a winter piece, however it can be worn in warmer winter climates with a suit.

Go all out for spring racing carnival as this is a great starting point to create a crazy 'loud' outfit. Pair your liberty print shirt with a windowpane check suit, knit tie, fun socks and a pair of brogues. Don't forget a loud pocket square and straw hat to complete the ensemble.

WHITE T-SHIRT

You will wear your white t-shirt until it dies, it is so versatile. I would recommend at least three classic white t-shirts in good working condition for your wardrobe. Wear your white t-shirts with casual shorts, chinos and denim, swimming trunks, anything really. For the adventurous, try paring it back with a cotton suit and sneakers.

Your t-shirts should be replaced every other summer as they lose their color and shape.

A point to think about—there is an age limit here or, more to the point, a fitness limit. If you have a less than trim physique, let go of the t-shirt. Opt for a loose fitting white shirt instead.

BLACK T-SHIRT

These are great for seeing live bands where you dance like a mad man and sweat up a storm. Great for kicking around on casual summer evenings with tan chinos and espadrilles for a coastal vibe.

DENIM SHIRT

Your partner will love denim on you; its sexy, gritty and masculine. Impress on your next night out with double denim or pair your denim shirt with black or olive green chinos. For the adventurous, try triple denim; shirt, jacket and jeans and different shades for a strong masculine American work wear look. My pick for triple denim is black jeans with a faded blue denim shirt and dark denim jacket.

DARK DENIM JEANS

Dark slim over-dyed denim jeans are a must for casual Friday, weekend casual and smart casual looks. Dark indigo and black are the first of your denim essentials closely followed by a washed back/burnished, lighter denim for the warmer months.

Go for the casual look here. Just add a pair of white sneakers and a t-shirt.

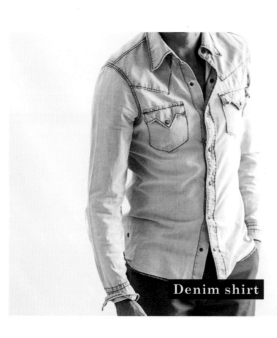

Denim shirt

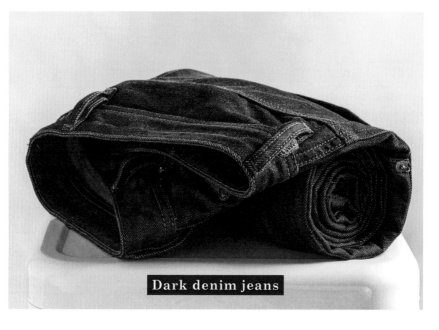

Dark denim jeans

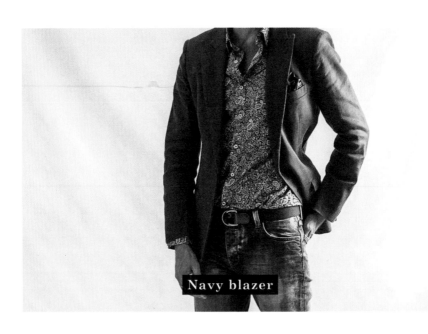

Navy blazer

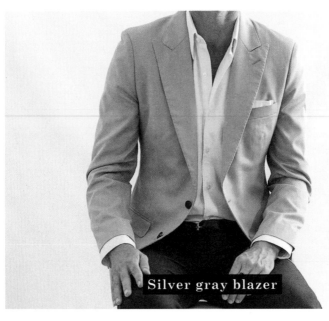

Silver gray blazer

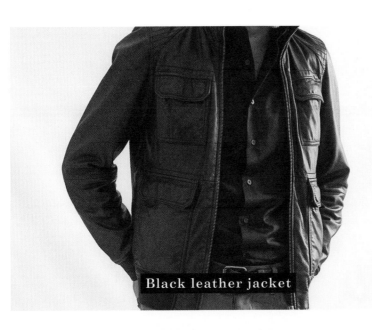

Black leather jacket

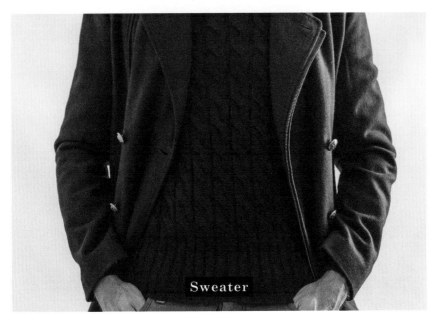

Sweater

Another smart casual combination that works is a woven shirt tucked in with a blazer, a canvas belt and loafers. Casual Friday at work is a little more styled with a pair of brogues and fun socks teamed up with a club or knit tie in addition to the smart casual combination above.

NAVY BLAZER

The jewel in the crown, the navy blazer is the ultimate utility piece. A well-fitted navy blazer works with t-shirts and jeans through to chinos and trousers and dress shirts.

This is a 'must have' wardrobe essential. Personally I like to have one Spring/Summer weight navy blazer and an Autumn/Winter weight navy blazer—that's how important this is for your smart casual wardrobe.

For the adventurous, try a navy blazer pared back with white denim jeans or trousers and white woven shirt or t-shirt.

SILVER GRAY BLAZER

A cotton or linen/cotton blazer for casual through to cocktail wear. Consider this look: team with dark trousers, white shirt, white pocket square, black derby shoes—perfect for cocktails.

Add a second wool version for Autumn/Winter. Tan trousers and a crisp white shirt with chocolate brown shoes and belt is a nice combination.

For the adventurous, try a black shirt back with white denim with your gray blazer in summer for a change at evening events.

BLACK LEATHER JACKET

There are two main types of black leather jackets: biker or bomber. Choose the biker look which is a grungier look, or the bomber jacket which is a tad more elegant. The shorter bomber style leather jacket is perfect for traveling.

Marlon Brando made it famous by just throwing on old jeans, a t-shirt and casual boots. You can too and away you go.

BEIGE TRENCH COAT

The length is extremely important to make this traditional piece work for you. Your trench coat can be worn for casual and business and for everything in between.

SWEATER

Navy merino fine wool sweater in a crew neck will serve you well when wearing chinos, jeans or smart tailored trousers. I like to use mine with separates like a tan chino with a navy check blazer.

For the adventurous, try your navy knit with white denim and striped espadrilles for springtime sailing.

PULLOVER

This piece will keep you warm and compliment dark or raw denim jeans with a pair of casual boots or sneakers.

A hoodie or crew neck pullover in a college motif (if it's a college that you actually attended for more than a day), print or plain light gray marl is best.

For the adventurous, try a black or navy gilet over the top with your favorite jeans and sneakers.

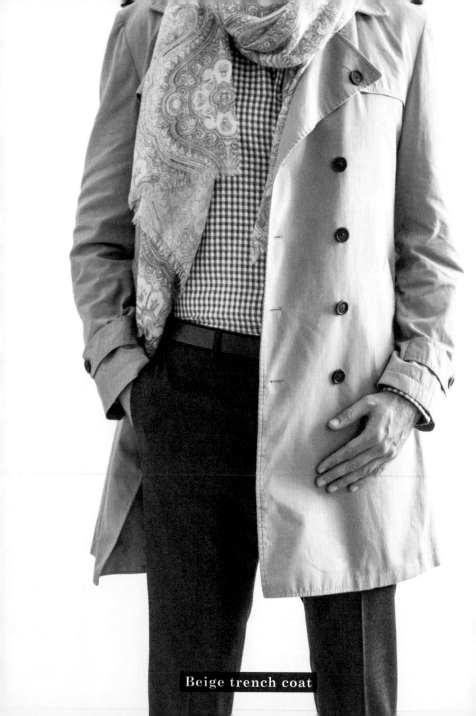

Beige trench coat

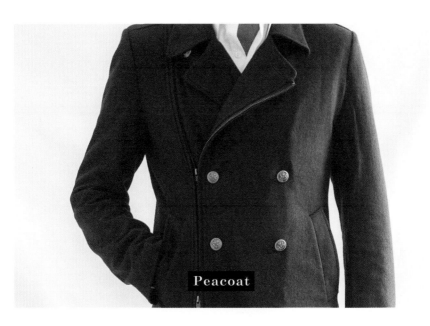

Peacoat

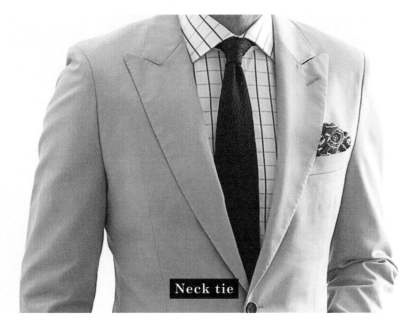

Neck tie

PEACOAT

Buy a quality wool coat and look after it and you'll have it forever. Buy once, buy right is definitely the motto here.

Look for a navy or charcoal double-breasted peacoat with contrast buttons. The quality of the buttons will make a huge difference to the finished look of the garment so look closely at the buttons. Make sure the length covers your backside.

TIES

A plain silver gray medium width tie won't go out of fashion too quickly and it creates a clever understated look. It would suit events such as weddings and funerals, awards and gala dinners. A club tie with a couple of colors in a stripe works for smart casual through to business wear.

BOW TIE

A traditional hand-tied bow tie in black with white dots is versatile and would cover all formal occasions. Play it safe with a plain black silk bow tie for summer and plain black velvet bow tie for winter. If you can't be bothered perfecting the hand tie, get an adjustable one and be sure it fits tight up into the collar, as they look terrible when loose.

WHITE POCKET SQUARE

This is a useful accessory for smart casual, business and formal occasions. Wear it as a knife sharp square or fluff it up into a 'fop' for some texture.

Perhaps choose a linen square for the knife sharp look and a silk option for the fop style.

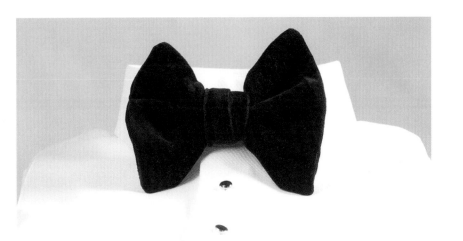

Bow tie

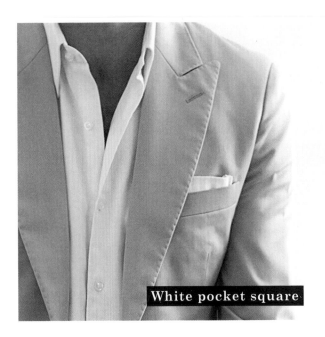

White pocket square

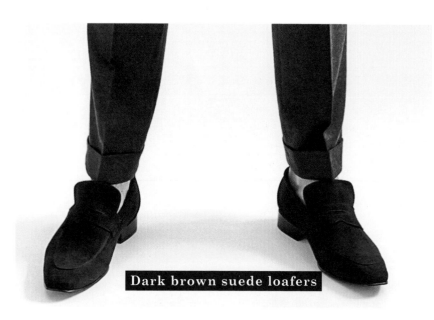

Dark brown suede loafers

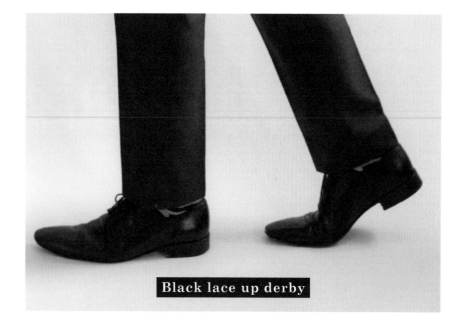

Black lace up derby

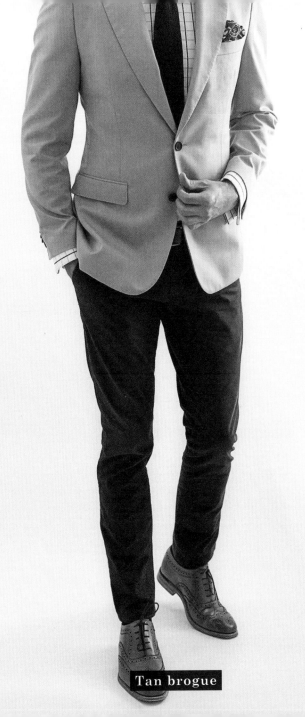

Tan brogue

DARK BROWN SUEDE LOAFERS

Team your suede loafers with shorts and a long sleeved linen shirt that will create a great casual outfit. Also try chinos or denim jeans with a casual cotton woven shirt or a t-shirt for a cool yet smart casual look.

Sans socks or hidden sockettes are the go. You do not want to show any sock of any variety. Loafers in leather with an antique finish are a nice option too.

BLACK LACE UP DERBY

For smart casual to business to cocktail and formal (if you don't have patent leather shoes), the black lace-up derby shoe is essential for your closet.

Traditionally a business shoe for suiting, this staple item can be dressed down as well to create a more relaxed look. Avoid wearing with chinos, as these shoes are too formal for such a casual look.

TAN BROGUE

A British classic, you can find the best hand-made versions from the top bespoke makers in Britain. The tan brogue is perfect with denim jeans and chinos paired with woven shirts and blazers.

Think about wearing these on casual Fridays at work or when meeting up with friends for a relaxed lunch. I would wear tan brogues with casual suiting—think cotton earth tones.

For the adventurous, pair them back with a light gray or steel blue suit, white shirt and navy tie for business.

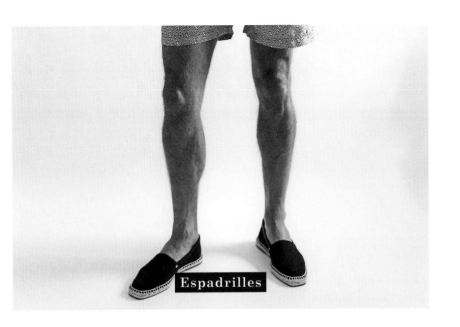

Espadrilles

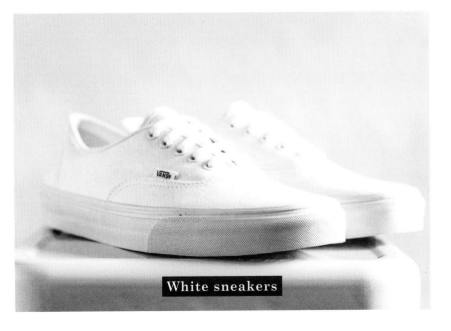

White sneakers

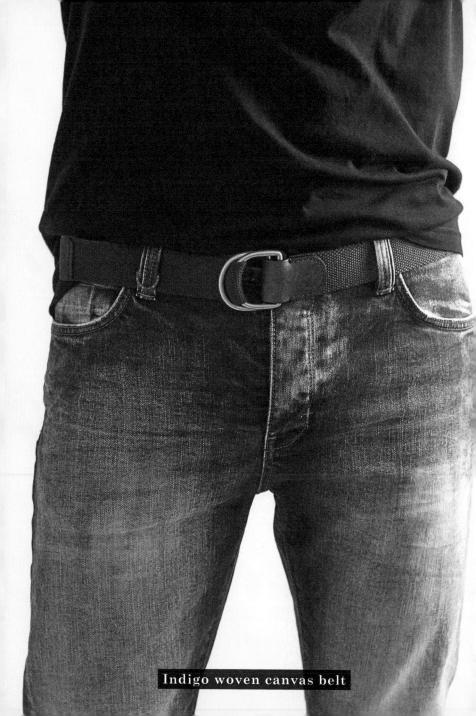

Indigo woven canvas belt

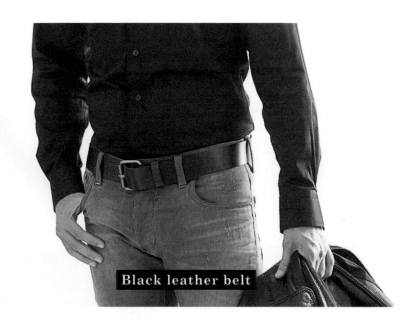

Black leather belt

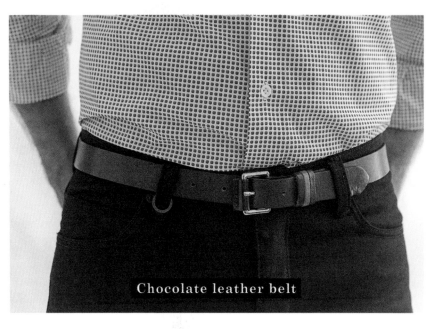

Chocolate leather belt

ESPADRILLES

For sailing, poolside and the beach, these are essential footwear. These bad boys are cool, comfortable and lightweight. Espadrilles are easy to wear but not terribly supportive, so don't expect to do too much walking in them.

Wear them with swimming trunks, shorts, rolled chinos and even beat-up faded denim. If worn regularly, you will most likely get one to two seasons out of them.

For the adventurous, try espadrilles with a cotton suit and t-shirt and finish with a panama hat.

Trade your thongs or flip-flops in on a pair of espadrilles—you won't go wrong.

WHITE SNEAKERS

For your classic white sneaker or sandshoe, consider brands such Converse, Vans or Lactose. Be sure to get some low-cut sockettes, as you don't want to show any signs of socks when you are wearing your sneakers with shorts, cropped denim and chinos. Throw them in the washing machine occasionally to keep them looking and smelling fresh. Limit their outings in winter to dry days only.

INDIGO WOVEN CANVAS BELT

This belt is essential with shorts, chinos and jeans. I wear my navy blue canvas belt with denim jeans and chinos as well as tailored shorts. My preference is 'o ring' or 'd ring' buckles for canvas belts.

My belt rule about color coordinating: try to match the shoes or match the pants.

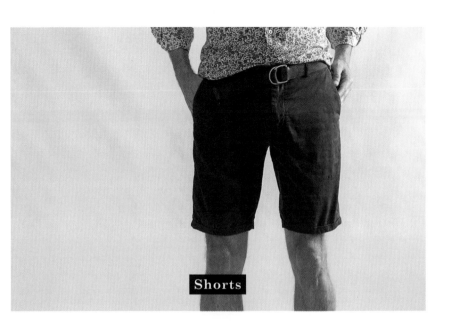

Shorts

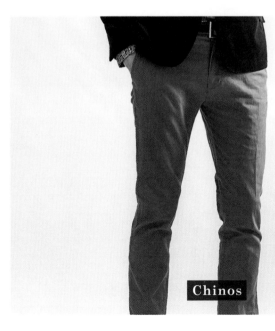

Chinos

TAN LEATHER PLAIT BELT

Choose a belt with no embellishments and a simple buckle. The width of your belt should sit comfortably in the boot loops of trousers and jeans.

The belt must match dress shoes as well as smart casual shoes.

BLACK LEATHER BELT

The same applies as for the plait belt above.

Choose a belt with no embellishments and a simple buckle. The width of your belt should sit comfortably in the boot loops of trousers and jeans.

Make sure the belt matches both dress and smart casual shoes.

CHOCOLATE LEATHER BELT

Ditto above. Choose a belt with no embellishments and a simple buckle.

The width of your belt should sit comfortably in the boot loops of trousers and jeans.

The belt must match dress shoes as well as smart casual shoes.

SHORTS

Tan, navy, white and a fashion color like olive green in a length that suits your body type.

Shorts should be balanced to your shape and height. The more details or embellishments on shorts, the faster they will date.

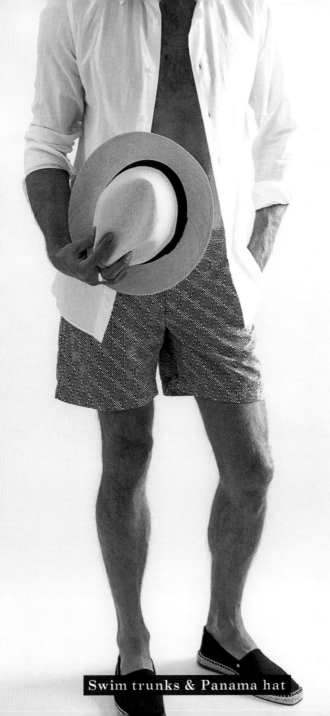

Swim trunks & Panama hat

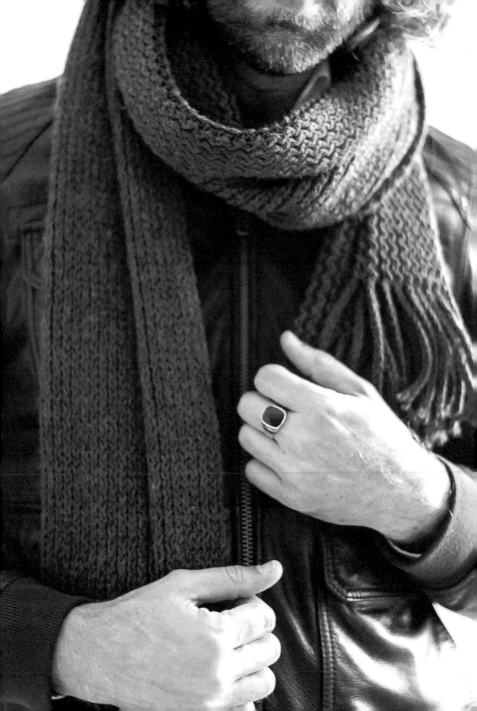

CHINOS

Navy, tan, olive green are the essential colors for year round casual trousers. Other colors like pink and cobalt may take be added to your wardrobe over and above your essentials.

A classic combination is tan chinos with a white shirt and navy blazer. For the adventurous, try navy chinos with a lightweight navy sweater with your favorite casual boots.

SWIM TRUNKS

Plain colored and a repetitive print in a suitable length for your body type.

PANAMA HAT

This summer essential is available in cream or tobacco. Wear with swim trunks and a loose linen shirt with espadrilles for boating or the beach. For a smart casual look, try chinos, woven shirt with blazer and loafers for the perfect Polo ensemble.

SCARF

A plain gray textured scarf is the most versatile color. A scarf with a fleck or tonal pattern would work also.

TAKEAWAYS

- Save up and invest in the big-ticket items for suits, coats and footwear.
- Buy once, buy right.
- Once you have these essentials, just build the areas of the wardrobe that get the most use.

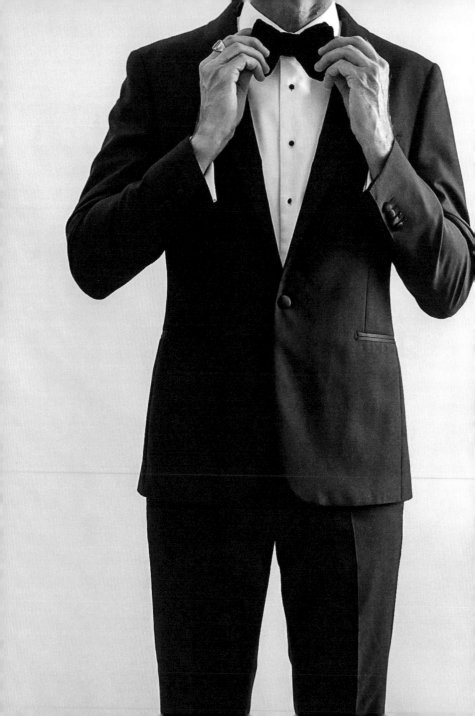

Chapter Eight

DECIPHER THE DRESS CODE

You have just received an invitation to an event and at the very bottom you can see a dress code. What does this mean?

If you have seen celebrities on the red carpet, you'll see that one person's interpretation of the dress code can be quite different from another's. Likewise I am sure you have rolled into a party and seen someone who was overdressed and someone who was underdressed.

My advice is to play it safe and adhere to the code.

A guide to dress codes

- *Black tie—tuxedo, white dinner shirt with a black bow tie is required. Black or midnight navy blue is the tuxedos of choice right now.*
  Accessories such as cuff links and shirt studs add polish.

*High shine or patent leather shoes are ideal, but velvet
is also an option for the adventurous. A dinner shirt
and bow tie is an inexpensive addition and well worth
having.*

- *Cocktail—black suit with white shirt and neck tie works.
  A velvet blazer for cooler weather is a nice option that
  can combine well with a pair of dark trousers.*

- *Lounge suit—traditionally, this means a single-breasted
  suit in navy, blues, gray or taupe with a shirt and tie.
  A vest is optional. A pocket square is a nice additional
  touch.*

- *Smart/business casual—single or double breasted blazer
  or sports coat with trousers or chinos, collared shirt in
  pale colors, stripes or gingham is the order of the day.
  No tie is required. Pocketed optional but no jeans.*

If you are going to a formal event, and you don't own a
tuxedo, a classic plain black suit will suffice.

Get your dress codes right and you'll feel confident for
any occasion.

TAKEAWAYS

- It shows respect for the host and guests when you follow the
  dress code.
- Build key event pieces into your wardrobe to give you some
  choice.
- When you can afford it, buy a classically-cut black tuxedo.

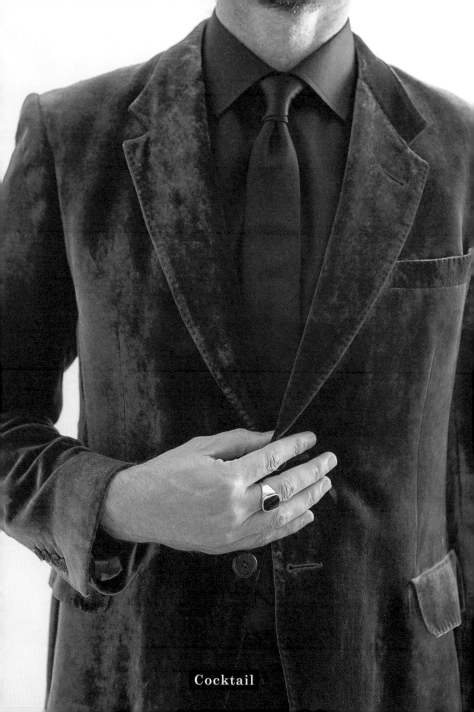

Cocktail

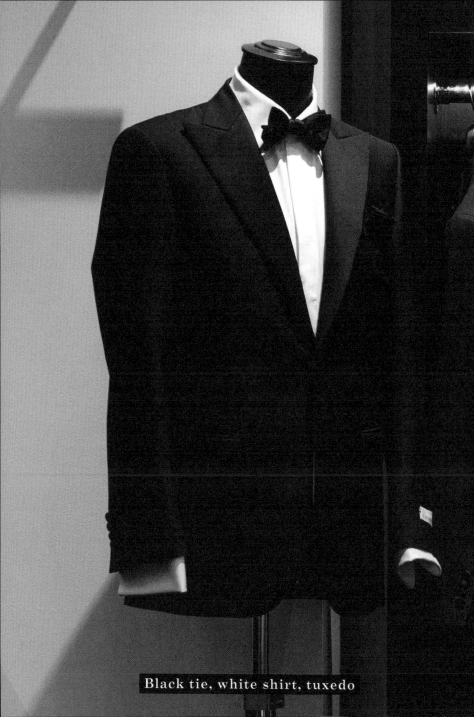

Black tie, white shirt, tuxedo

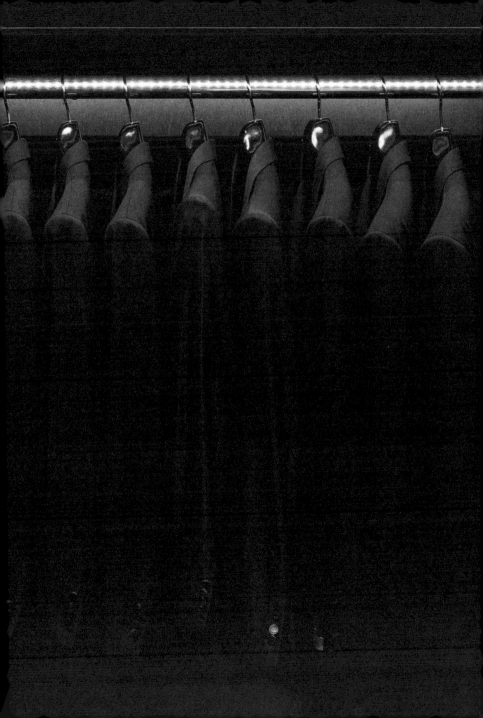

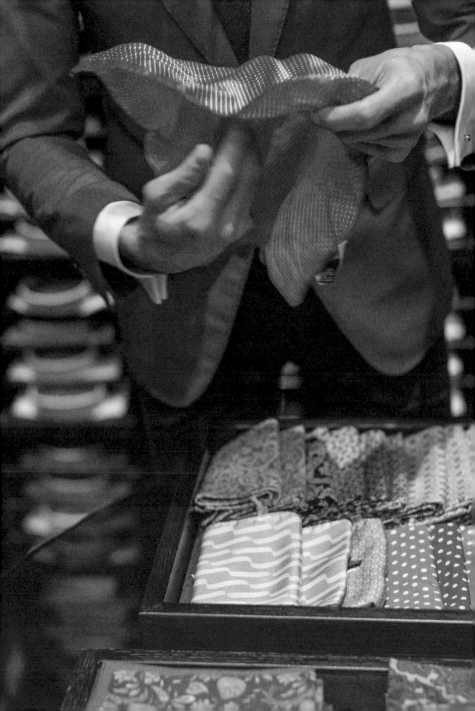

ACCESSORY TO THE FACT

How do you accessorize without looking 'overly styled'?

Accessories can literally make or break an outfit. You can put together a spectacular ensemble but without accessories, it just seems to be missing that special something.

Keeping to the minimalist theme of this book, careful consideration is needed when selecting, styling and wearing accessories.

A guide to accessorizing

- *A tie adds a touch of personality to a shirt and the knot and length of the tie are crucial to making a great impact on your ensemble. Textured ties in linen, silk knits and wool make for a nice change from your regular silk ties.*

- *A pocket square adds class and sophistication to a suit. You don't need to match with your ties any more, but you would do well to coordinate the pocket square with the tie or the shirt. Wear as a knife sharp square or fluff it up into a 'fop'.*
- *Colored socks brighten up business shoes and tell your audience that you have a little sass, some drive and ambition. Your colored socks don't need to be patterned as well, but you can mix up classic, block and fancy socks for a full compliment of choice.*
- *Cuff links finish off cuffs. Even though this trend is past its peak, if done elegantly, cuff links are timeless. Real metals and real stones are the way to go. If you have a watch, consider coordinating the look of these two pieces.*
- *A tie bar is functional and provides flair. It is best suited to clean classic suits and only really works if the entire outfit is well put together. If you wear a tie bar with a poorly knotted tie, or if you look disheveled, the effect will be completely lost.*
- *Scarves cannot only keep you warm but are a brilliant way to add texture to an outfit and hide extra weight.*
- *Bags are definitely more than just a carry all and for the modern gent, an accessory that contributes to your personal style. Backpacks, satchels, gym bags and weekenders can all play a part in the modern gent's wardrobe and life. When buying leather bags, be sure to get a generic color as they last a long time and coordinate well with classic footwear.*
- *Hats are super trendy, functional and always stylish. Get a shape that suits your face in a color that suits your*

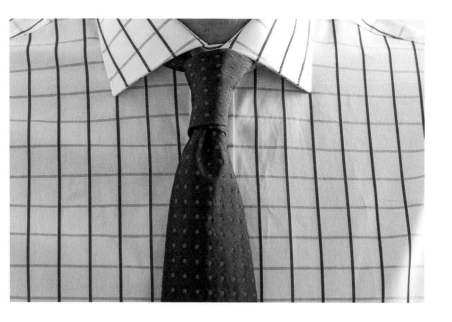

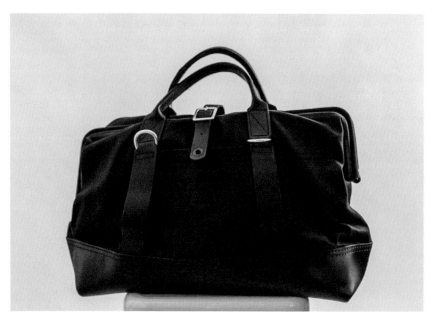

hair and skin tone with a brim that suits your stature.

- *Jewelry is easy to get wrong, but when executed tastefully, it brings soul and balance to a look.*

- *Glasses and sunglasses frame the face and can really add style to your personal brand. Check out the chapter 'Framed'.*

- *One signature ring is something that can be worn with anything to any event. Buy once, buy right, and pass it on to future family members.*

- *A minimal cluster of bangles is like a badge of honor for the modern gentleman.*

- *A watch is extremely potent in your accessories game. It tells your audience about your taste, your lifestyle and your commitment to an investment piece. Take your time in making this purchase and spend as much as you can afford to get this integral piece right. Once you have one timepiece, there is no reason not to keep building more into your wardrobe.*

- *A chain is either rock n' roll or sleazy, so choose wisely. The biggest issues are—you can look a little 'try hard' or at the other end of the spectrum, a little effeminate. It may be safe just to leave this area alone.*

Modern accessorizing is about 'a little less is more'. Don't put every accessory you own on at the same time. It can be distracting and lacks direction.

Wearing lots of accessories takes away from the overall image and message you want to portray—again, less is more. Accessories should accentuate your personality not distract from it .

Jewelry is best when it has a back story, handed down through family, vintage or from that trip to Rome. The significance of a piece will also give you pride in your appearance.

TAKEAWAYS

- Less is more when it comes to accessories.
- Minimal is still the theme here.
- Purchase or acquire pieces with meaning.
- Accentuate your personality with carefully chosen accessories.

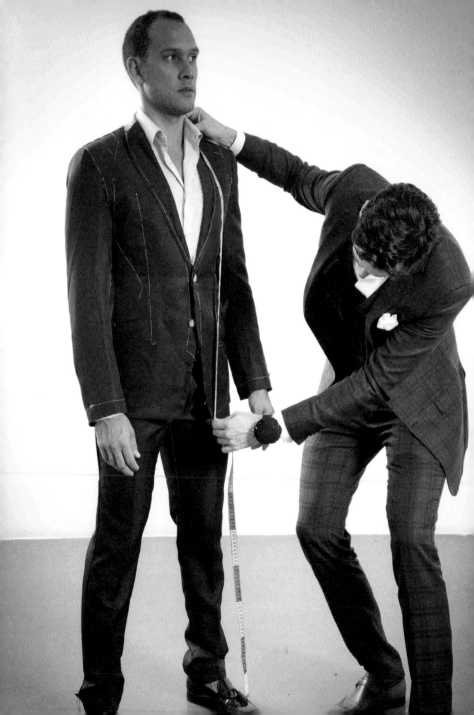

Chapter Ten

BESPOKE

What is bespoke and why should you try it?

Not to be confused with made to measure, bespoke is hand-made—something made specifically for you, in the fabric you choose and to your particular measurements.

Every man should try the bespoke experience at least once. Perhaps start with having a shirt made, then if you like it move to ties, shoes and suits.

A bespoke suit can take around 40 hours to make. This is living breathing work by a true artisan. Centuries of tailoring are behind these hand-crafted pieces and today we are blessed with the most dynamic comfortable suits history has ever seen. Suits can be worn for work, play and everyday.

I have seen loads of amazing tailoring from all around the world: Italy, France, the UK, the US, Australia and throughout Asia. So, you'll most likely find an excellent local tailor near you.

To achieve a great result, two or three fittings are required—of course, this option is not available if you are measured remotely. Choosing the right cloth is vital for a great result. Fine fitting and construction will be let down by rubbish fabrics that don't sit, wear or last well. My recommendation is to find a reputable local tailor known for quality fabrics and service so you can be involved in every step.

BESPOKE SHIRTS

It's all well and good to wear the latest fashion, but let me ask you this—are you wearing fashion or is fashion wearing you? For example, I am tall with an average to long neck and can wear most styles of shirt collars. If I choose to wear a smaller 'beatnik' 60s collar, this makes my neck look bigger. If I wear a larger 70s style collar with a tall collar stand, my neck looks remarkably smaller. And as you can imagine, something in between is just about right. All three styles are available now, so how do you figure which one is right for you? Consider these three important things when choosing your next bespoke shirt—fabric, fit, style.

The right fabric

Fabric choice is the most difficult part of the process, however it is very rewarding when you choose well and you see a swatch that will become a perfectly fitted shirt.

Are you tactile? Perhaps a shirt with texture, a self-stripe or herringbone may have a nice feel about it that floats your boat. Do you feel the heat? Perhaps lightweight pure cotton is right for you. Do you iron your own shirts? Maybe a little elestane or polyester in with your cotton shirt will make life a little easier.

In terms of color, I believe every man should have black, white, navy and lilac shirts in their wardrobe. These colors cover the key events in your life. Black is sexy and a great evening shirt to wear on a date or out to dinner. White is incredibly versatile and can be worn to just about every occasion. Consider having at least a few white shirts. Navy is flattering and brilliant with a pair of jeans or chinos. Lilac is a fantastic color for corporate business as it's welcoming and works well with every skin tone.

The right fit

Bespoke is all about getting well fitted shirts. All bodies were not created equal so why should we have to make do with 'off the rack' shirts? With bespoke shirts, body length and width, sleeves, cuffs and collar are tailored to fit your unique body type.

Look to balance the collar shape with your neck as mentioned earlier. Be certain to have the length of your shirt proportionate to how you will wear it. Add a little extra room for your watch and a finger space should fit comfortably inside the collar when fastened. Your favorite shirt will be the one that feels best—that invariably comes from a perfect fit.

The right style

When ordering your bespoke shirt, think about what will work for you. What are you comfortable wearing? Your tailor will help you when choosing fabric and fit to suit you.

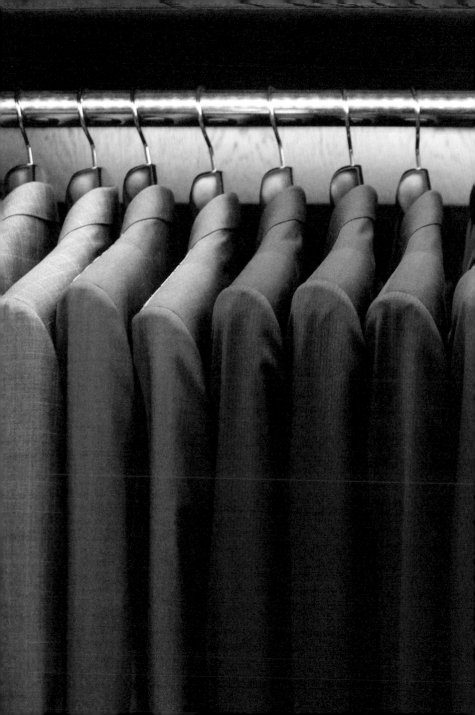

BESPOKE SUITS

This is, hands down, the best shopping experience you will ever have. The decision to spend more money on a piece of clothing than you ever have in the past, the initial appointment, selecting the fabric and style, going to all the fittings. It's very empowering. This is a time-honored tradition that was passed down through the ages. In the 21st century bespoke is becoming more prevalent than it has been in the last 20 years or so.

Young men in their first jobs are investing in a bespoke suit as they see it paying off in the long run. The earlier you start, the sooner your personal style will become evident. We live in a technological age where getting ahead just cannot happen quickly enough. Every edge you have over your competition is a bonus.

Why bother with a bespoke suit? It makes a statement in the corporate environment where others look like they have come out of a cookie cutter. A bespoke wedding suit for the perfect wedding look will stand the test of time. (Who am I kidding, all wedding photos look hilarious in ten years time!) The point is at the time it was perfect and you had a ball.

So what are the pitfalls of buying bespoke? The decisions are yours and it can be easy to be talked into something you are not sure about, just like when shopping retail. Whiskey is often consumed as part of the tradition of ordering bespoke. Try to hold out until you have made the most important decisions. It's an investment, so choose wisely. You want all of your investments to pay dividends and the best way to safeguard this particular investment is to take things slowly. Approach this project with patience and clarity. Do your due diligence and share your inspiration with your tailor.

What are the benefits of buying bespoke? The feeling of clothing that just fits perfectly is an absolute treat. Your peers will notice and so will potential partners. Having your unique style etched on the finer details of your suit makes it uniquely yours and this allows you to be your authentic self.

Getting your bespoke suit made

Find a tailor. You may get recommendations for a good tailor from mates and colleagues. It's best that you like the look of the completed work, not just a verbal endorsement, as all men tend to believe their tailor is the best.

Find your style. Do your due diligence, research Tumblr, Instagram, Facebook and the web to find the looks that appeal to you most. Collate these findings and take them to your initial consultation.

Meet your tailor. In this meeting you can work out the design for your suit, be measured, and place your order which will require a deposit.

Alternatively, you can just cover off on design elements like fabric, buttons, and stitching, internal construction and come back after you have considered the design. In this scenario, you will be measured at this second meeting.

The tailor will ask questions to make sure you get what you want and need. He'll want to know where and when the suit will be worn. Is it for work or an event? Is it worn year round or just during one season?

Ask, as many questions as you can think of. There is no such thing as a silly question when it comes to this personal investment. Also if you have a history of wearing through parts of your trousers or jackets, this needs to be covered off, as parts of the suit can be made stronger to endure the pressures of your everyday life.

Attend the first fitting. This is where the tailor fits the baste to your body. It's the basic internal construction without any finishing touches, like lining and treatments. The tailor will usually use chalk to mark changes to anything that you both agree to. You need to speak up about how the suit feels in this part of the fitting process. The tailor may want you back for fitting during the construction or not as the case may be.

Attend the final fitting. This is where the hard work comes to life. What was in your mind's eye, you are now wearing. Hallelujah, it fits! This is your last opportunity to make any tiny, final adjustments and pay the creative legend your final payment. Have a chat about styling the suit, what shirts, shoes and ties coordinate well. Pocket squares, collar pins, cuff links and tie bars can be selected to finish off your brand new work of art.

Wear the damn thing to death! Having a bespoke suit that comes out for a play once a year is an absolute waste in my books. Yes, it was more than you ordinarily pay for a suit. Yes, it is special, but its been designed and manufactured to be worn to impress, for you to look and feel good in. Your new bespoke suit will change your life so wear it and enjoy.

BESPOKE SHOES

I can spot ill-fitting shoes a country mile away. They bulge out at the sides. There are gaps in the heel cup or deep folds across the bridge. All are signs your shoes are not fitting you as well as they should. We have all had shoes that look good but are just too uncomfortable to spend long periods of time in. Shoes can impact on your knees, hips and back so take your shoes seriously. My gramps said, "Look after your back and your feet son." That's what bespoke shoes do.

The process is straight forward when ordering bespoke shoes—and a little less time consuming than having a shirt, suit or blazer fitted.

Steps to getting bespoke shoes made

- *Find a cobbler.*
- *Measure feet.*
- *Find a block that suits.*
- *Choose the leather.*
- *Choose the color.*
- *Choose the finish.*
- *Wait a month for your fitting.*
- *Final tweaks are made if required.*
- *Boom! Walk like an Egyptian.*

BESPOKE TIES

Bespoke obviously caters for hard-to-fit gents who can't get a good fit with off-the-rack apparel—ties are no exception. Tall gents such as myself need an extra long tie so the tail isn't too short and shorter gents need a tail that is shorter.

Here is how you can check to see if bespoke is for you.

Tie your favorite knot and see where the tail of the tie ends, if it doesn't tuck in behind the front part of the tie, then it is too short. If it's longer than the front part of the tie, it's too long. Bespoke ties are made by tailors so rock up at your favorite tailor, choose a fabric that suits you in a length and width that suits you best. Easy!

TAKEAWAYS

■ Bespoke is an experience you won't forget all for the right reasons.

■ You will be proud to wear the pieces you have had a hand in designing.

■ There is no substitute for good quality and great cut.

■ You will look good and feel great.

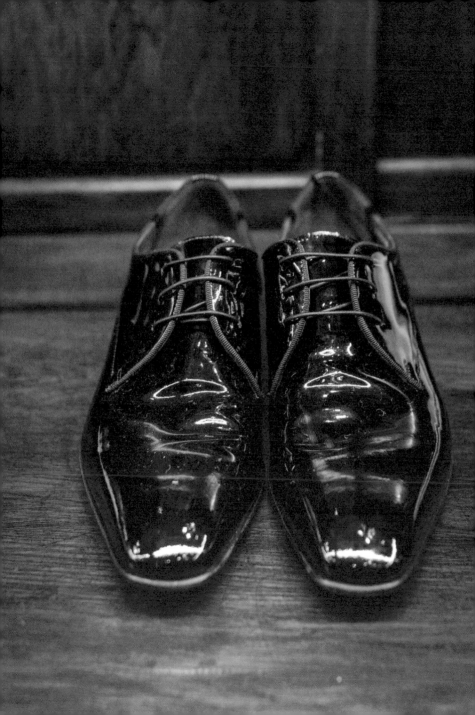

Chapter Eleven

WELL HEELED

The first thing to know about footwear—buy quality shoes because they will last longer and they'll be more comfortable.

In saying that, what does your footwear say about you? First impressions are important. Footwear can make or break an outfit. How does your footwear fare?

How is the condition and presentation of your footwear? If your shoes are in poor condition, it will ruin the whole effect of your ensemble. You will be noticed for the wrong reasons. Being well shod, people may not notice your footwear because the total effect is simply one of excellence. Wearing the right footwear for an occasion is important.

A guide to what shoes to wear
- *Sneakers are perfect for casual, ready to run, fun, carefree days.*
- *High tops are great for basketball and other sports, dancing, DJing and being a cool cat.*

- *Loafers when you want to be smooth, sophisticated and elegant.*
- *Brogues are for the traditional, sensible you with a cool modern edge.*
- *Desert boots show your practical but contemporary side, that you are a can do guy.*
- *Military boots for when you don't mind getting dirty— functional and tough.*

There is also a grungy, antique or vintage vibe in so many ensembles these days that what may appear to the untrained eye as sloppy or disheveled is in fact quite deliberate. The music industry has always had an influence over what to wear and footwear is no exception.

You'll see high tops in hip hop, mountain/military boots in folk and rock, desert boots in Indy and sneakers in electronic music. These are not hard and fast rules—just an observation.

Your choice of footwear can profoundly impact on your overall look. Mixing up styles can create something completely different.

Sneakers with a suit for example will make the outfit more relaxed and fun, whereas when paired with an oxford or derby shoe, the suit ensemble looks sharp and sophisticated.

Throw on a pair of beaten up well-worn brogues with tailored shorts and a loose linen shirt and it's smart casual. Wearing a pair of espadrilles will give this ensemble a beach or boating vibe.

Mix things up a bit. For example, I love my blue velvet

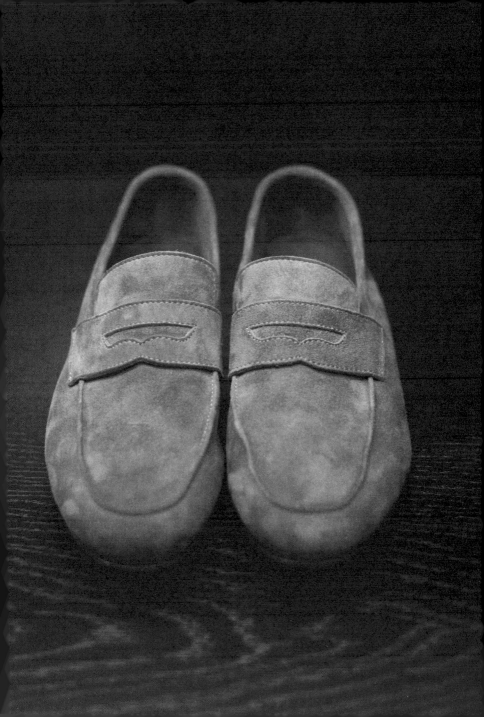

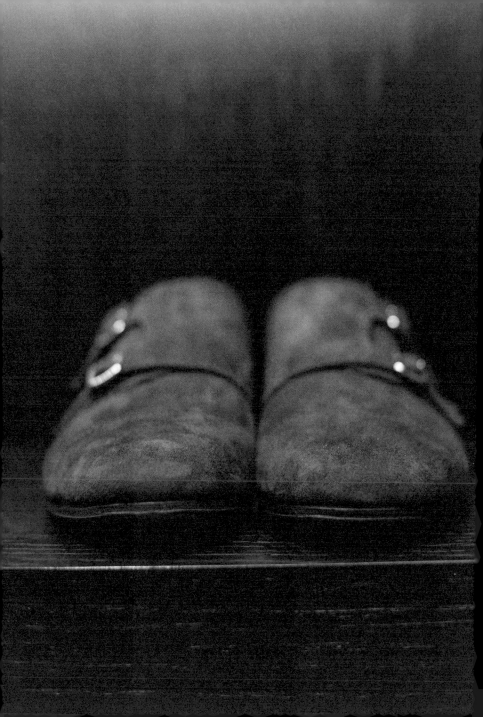

slippers with denim jeans and a casual shirt. Mixing up the genres using different footwear choices can be difficult but executed well, it can really have your mates jealous of your styling prowess and confidence.

The fact is, the more types of shoes you have in your wardrobe, the easier your styling becomes and the more options you have to create unique authentic looks. You'll be pleasantly surprised with the outcome.

TAKEAWAYS

- Good shoes can make an outfit.
- Quality shoes feel more comfortable and last longer.
- Make sure you have the right shoes for your different personas.
- There is no such thing as too many.

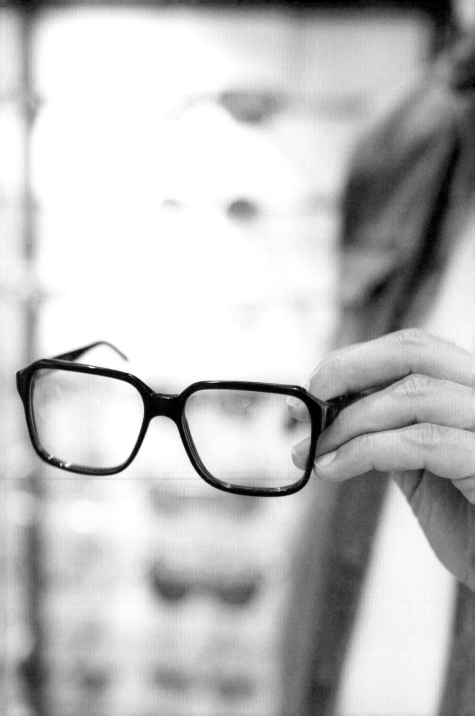

Chapter Twelve

FRAMED

Glasses can give a gent an air of cool intelligence and importance. They can also be essential for seeing.

Need new sunglasses or glasses? How do you work out what style suits you best? Do you have frames that you don't really like. Are you stuck in a rut when it comes to your eyewear? When it comes to choosing the right frames for your face, whether glasses or sunglasses, experiment in the store to work out which ones look best and why.

When selecting new glasses, your face shape, length, width and features all count. Balance and symmetry are the mainstays of choosing the right shaped frames.

Ensure that the style and color of your glasses works to enhance your best features. If you have blue eyes, consider a frame color that works to bring out the blue of your eyes. The frame should contrast with your face shape and fit the scale of your face.

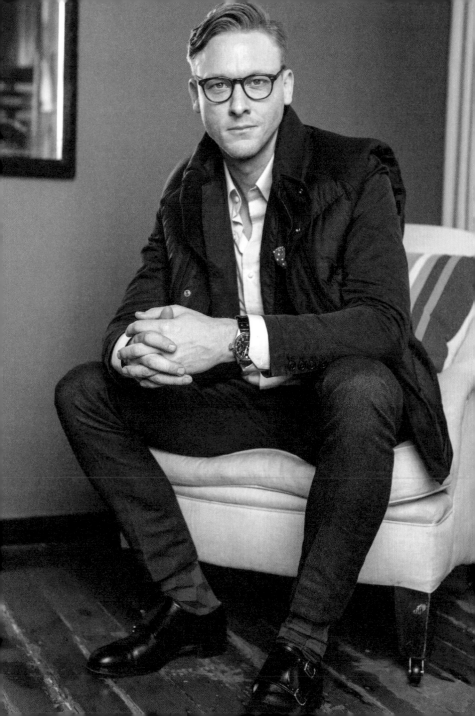

Guide for choosing frames on face shapes

- *If you have a round face, try angular narrow frames to lengthen your face.*
- *For an oval face, choose frames that are as wide as the broadest part of your face.*
- *For an oblong face, try a frame that has more depth than width.*
- *For a square shaped face, consider narrow frame styles with more width than depth or narrow oval shaped glasses.*
- *Base-down triangular face, look at frames that have strong features at the top of the frames to emphasize the upper third of your face.*
- *Base-up triangle (wide top, narrow bottom third of your face), light colored frames or rimless will work well.*
- *Diamond shape face: try frames with detailed or distinctive brow lines.*

Your hair color should also be taken into consideration when thinking about colors in your frames. Your face and skin coloring are unique. Most skin colorings tend to be blue (cool) or yellow (warm). Determine what your skin tone is. For blue cool tones, choose frames that are gray, pink, blue, plum, rose, jade, coal or amethyst. For warm skin tones, red, tortoise, copper, cream, khaki, beige, orange can work well. For the adventurous, break the rules and try more exaggerated styles.

Eyewear has always been dictated by fashion trends. The heavier retro look that Tom Ford and Oliver Peoples have going is very much a 70s vibe. Then there are the styles with finer rims coming in as the market and fashion change.

Take enough time to be interviewed by the optometrist and specialists in the store as it's a big decision and not to be taken lightly.

Most frames can't be adjusted, so you may find a fantastic frame that doesn't sit on the bridge of your nose properly and you will need to go back to the drawing board.

You really have to try on lots of pairs. Then cull to two or three, then down to one pair. It is a slow, gradual process for you to arrive at the finished product. Don't be afraid to have more than one consultation with your optometrist.

Just like building your wardrobe, your personal style is a reflection of your personality and your glasses frames are a big deal. Frames are the ultimate accessory that can be changed as often as your shoes—if that's your style. There really is no need to limit yourself when it comes to your options for your daily look.

TAKEAWAYS

- Get professional assistance.
- Try on lots of pairs.
- Take your time to make your decision and document the best two pairs that you find.
- Once you have the perfect pair, consider an additional pair for other parts of your lifestyle.
- Don't leave your glasses on top of your head as they will stretch and it just looks silly.

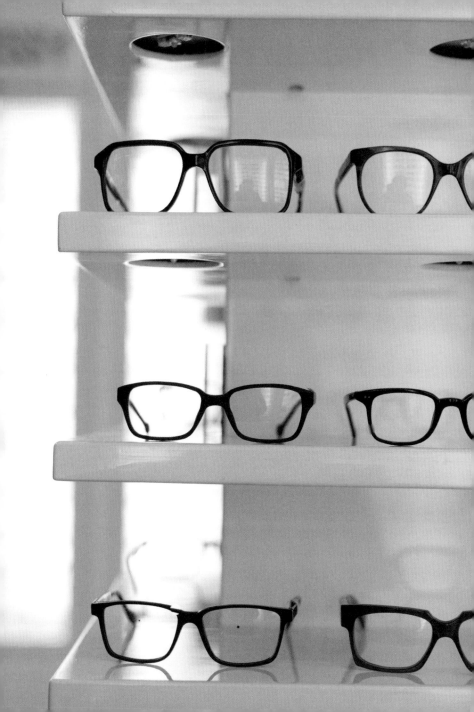

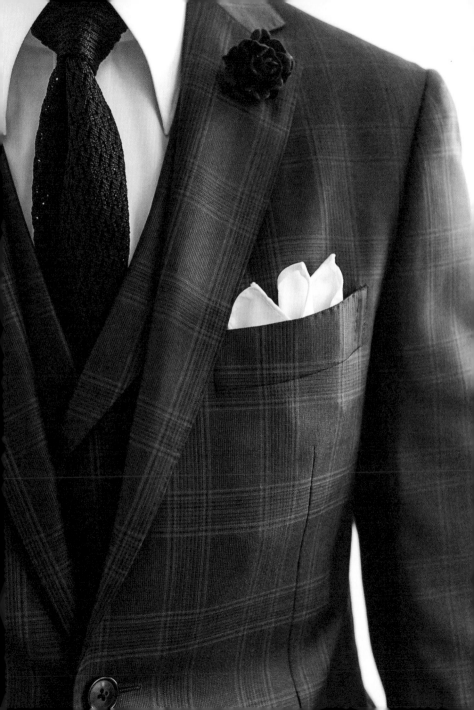

Chapter Thirteen

IT'S BUSINESS TIME

You spend the major part of your life working, so how is this fact represented in your wardrobe? Are you a corporate guy or a creative guy?

Whatever work you do, your business wardrobe is not a set uniform even if, in many ways, it sometimes feels like it is. Business socks, business shirts, business suits, business casual—it's all about looking 'the business'.

Here's some ideas for 'the basics' (for a two-week period) and how to build your ensembles for business from the '32 wardrobe essentials' in Chapter 7.

Corporate business wardrobe basics

- *3 suits*
- *10 business shirts*
- *10 ties*
- *5 pocket squares, mix of plain and patterned*
- *2 derby shoes—black and dark brown*
- *2 belts—black and dark brown*
- *10 socks—5 black and a mix of 5 patterned and plain*
- *1 tie bar*
- *1 lapel pin*
- *peacoat and scarf for winter*

Creative business wardrobe basics

- *2 denim—one dark and one light washed*
- *1 pair white or colored sneakers*
- *10 fun socks*
- *2 canvas belts*
- *8 printed, checks or striped shirts*
- *4 basic plain colored t-shirts*
- *2 casual cotton/linen blazers—one light color and one dark color*
- *1 tan brogues*
- *1 dark brown suede boots*
- *1 pair loafers*
- *1 double monk straps*
- *2 knit ties*
- *2 denim shirts—one dark and one washed-out colors*
- *1 peacoat*
- *1 scarf*
- *2 chinos—navy and tan*

CONTEMPORARY BUSINESS LOOK

The 3-piece suit is back. Waistcoats not only look smart but can also be very slimming. Depending on the cloth, the waistcoat can also make its way into your smart casual wardrobe. I like to mix up my 3-piece suit with denim instead of the matching trousers pared back with an open neck shirt and pocket square.

Separates (non-matching tops and bottoms) are back in a big way. What have been called 'sports coats and slacks' in the 80s are now 'trousers and blazers' in the 21st century. Combinations that are sympathetic to that previous era are a clean, modern, classic look that works brilliantly now.

The separate pieces (top and bottom) can be the same fabric (think cotton on cotton and wool on wool) but in modern classic cuts. Think large checks, windowpane and Prince of Wales check, paired back with block colored trousers and shirts.

Textured ties in wool and linen as well as silk knits with tie bars, collar pins, pocket squares and lapel pins all add to the peacock flair of the modern separates story.

Double-breasted blazers look awesome pared back with powdery mid-colored chinos in blue and green. Loud or fun socks tie the overall look together for a subtle, subdued ensemble.

To create a really smart ensemble, try blending a plain trouser in one of the colors in a check blazer. Add a neutral shirt, white or blue.

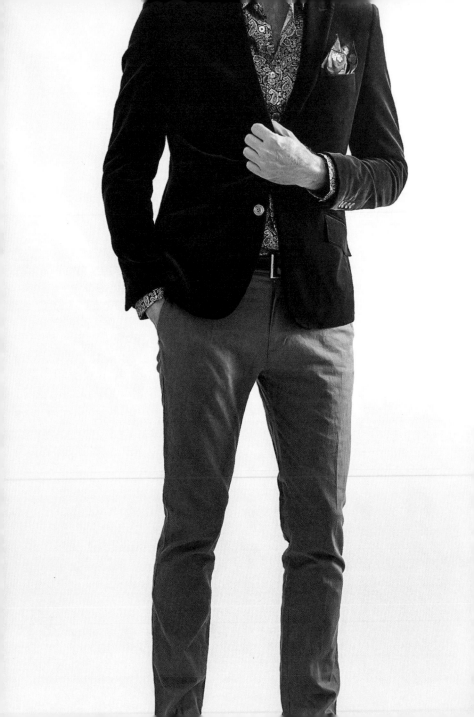

CASUAL FRIDAY

Does your workplace have dress down day or 'Casual Friday'?

It's a contentious issue and many employers worldwide cringe when they hear the term, Casual Friday. Others embrace the chance to wear some comfortable casual gear. Whatever you think, it can be really difficulty in deciphering what is appropriate to wear.

I like to think of this day as 'Fashion Friday'. Think about wearing an outfit that still looks stylish. This is an opportunity to impress so take the opportunity to wear something more creative.

If you are meeting clients when dressing down, make sure you still represent the authentic you and the business that you work in?

Think separates. Ask yourself, "Will this look be appropriate if I go to a bar or restaurant after work in the same outfit?"

Keep it real, keep it fun, don't slip into overall casual mode, keep your personal brand front and center.

TAKEAWAYS

- ■ Your business wardrobe is all about looking 'the business'.
- ■ Your business wardrobe makes up the major part of your overall wardrobe.
- ■ Casual Friday is not really that casual—make an effort.
- ■ Business casual is a no tie zone.
- ■ Mix and match for a contemporary business look.

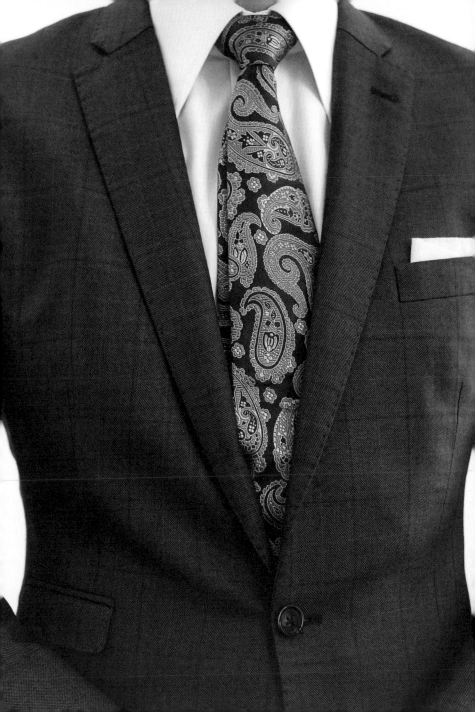

Chapter Fourteen

WHAT TO WEAR TO AN INTERVIEW

How do you nail the perfect look for an interview?

For a start, have a look at other chapters in this book: Credibility; Fit, Color, Style; It's Business Time; Routine Grooming; 32 Wardrobe Essentials.

When it comes to an interview, you are making a first impression. You really want your personal style to be strong and clear in this space. This is the case if you go to a second or third interview.

Business interviews can be daunting so having the right outfit on can reduce your stress and allow you to focus on the context of the meeting.

What to wear for a corporate interview

It is better to be overdressed for this occasion than underdressed. It's easy to take off a jacket in an interview after the greetings if you look too overdressed, but you can't pull one out if you didn't bring it.

Wearing a smart outfit with a suit as a base is where to start. A crisp white shirt is the best compliment to the suit. Dark brown or black lace up derby shoes with matching belt and a pair of navy socks that match the suit, anchors the ensemble.

Depending on the industry, you can add a pocket square and leave the shirt open or add a tie. Remember not to be over styled as this is distracting. You want to be engaging and impressive with your message and manner.

I have a friend who buys a new crisp white shirt every time he has a new speaking engagement, as he believes in perfect presentation and doesn't like to leave anything to chance.

Go for a contemporary look

In my experience styling creative clients, it is essential that you have a contemporary look to fit in with the industry custom. Let's start with a navy blazer and pare back with a pair of well-cut slim denim jeans. The shirt can be plain but it could also be a liberty print, checked or striped shirt for this important meeting. Brogues, fun socks and a canvas belt that doesn't really need to match, but must coordinate, is a great finish to this ensemble.

TAKEAWAYS

- Create a great first impression (and second and third).
- Think about a classic, simple, smart ensemble for your corporate interview.
- A blazer pared back with denim jeans is great for creative interviews.
- Don't over style it.
- A new white shirt will work every time.
- If you look good, you feel great.

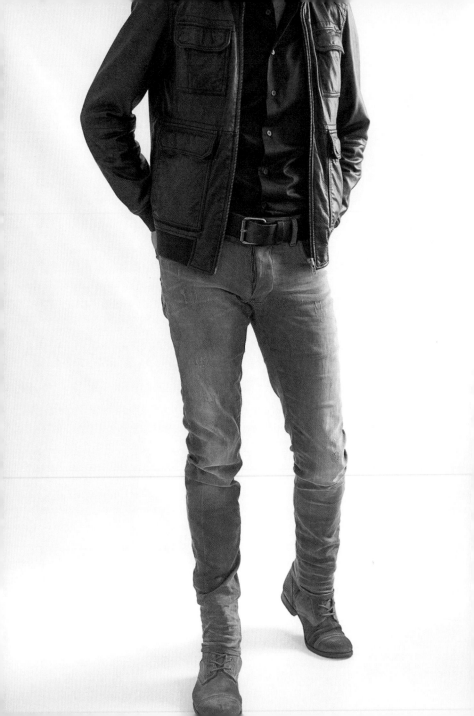

Chapter Fifteen

LOSE TEN POUNDS OFF YOUR LOOK

Everyone, regardless of their size, can look slimmer if they dress the right way. Tall, short, slim, robust we are all different. The following techniques I use everyday to style clients and myself.

In order to take ten pounds off your look, it's important to understand your unique fit, color and style. Most men tend to wear clothing that is too big for their actual size. A lot of men believe that hiding under bigger clothing helps, however this is not the case. The fit of your clothing is paramount to creating a slimmer looking shape.

Your fit lines are the finishes that work to make your

body shape look good. Neck line, waist line, hem lines for your jacket length, sleeve length and trouser length must be fitted correctly in order to show off your best features and draw attention away from less flattering areas. Anyone can make an Armani suit look bad if it doesn't fit properly.

I think most people know that black is the most slimming color, however navy and charcoal are also adequate slimming colors if black is too harsh against your skin tone.

Your hair, skin and eye color make up your unique look. Lighter colored eyes are a great place to start when finding colors that really suit you. Using your hair tone in accessories works well. Just like your unique body shape, there is no 'cookie cutter' solution for your colors.

Last but by no means least is style; this is how you wear your personality literally on your sleeve (if you are wearing sleeves). Show a little of your personality through your personal style to give a more accurate, non-verbal great first impression. Your posture and demeanor are better when you show your true personal style and this will create a slimmer and more confident image.

Think about how you can add some of your lifestyle and personality to your outfits through color with accessories to style yourself and your combinations.

Styling techniques to lengthen your overall look

- *Tucked in shirts create a halfway point or equator, this is balanced and slimming whereas un-tucked shirts can shorten your legs and overall look.*
- *Try contrasting colors to balance a shorter gentlemen for example: lighter bottoms with darker tops; for taller*

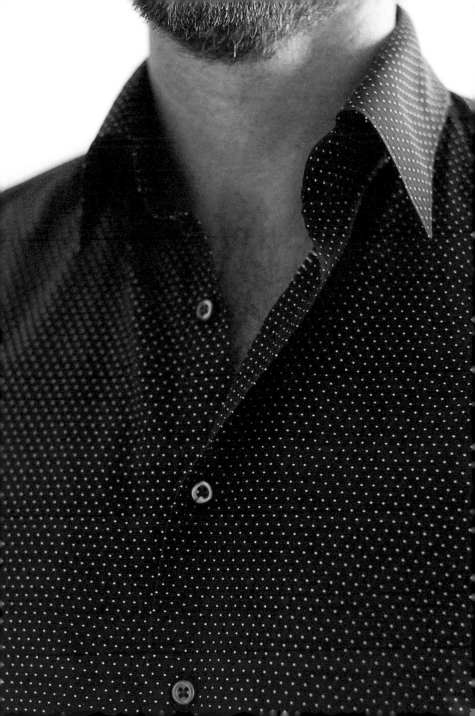

gents the opposite dark bottoms and lighter tops.

- *Leave the top two buttons on your shirt open to show skin to give the impression of length—it's why we don't trap the neckline by doing up the second button.*
- *Narrow finished hems will lengthen your look whereas wide finished hems will shorten.*
- *Pointed or longer shaped shoes can give a taller look as the round or block toe finishes are shortening, for example a tall slim guy throws on a pointed toe shoe this will make him look even taller than he actually is. Heavier thick type soles on these shoes can also make you look shorter and wider in spite of the extra height.*
- *A lighter colored shoe for the shorter gents draws attention to your feet and in turn lengthens your look.*
- *For taller gents looking to reduce overall height, try a darker shoe with darker bottoms to not draw any attention to your length.*

What to avoid

- *If your outfit is sprayed on (too tight) you will accentuate your weight—avoid at all costs.*
- *If your clothes are too baggy, you will look bigger than you actually are.*
- *If the hemlines are too long, this will shorten and likewise if the hems are too short, you will appear lanky. This applies to jacket length and sleeves on jackets.*

When I had the privilege of working with weight-loss contestants on the *Biggest Loser*, I could see my work come to life in a spectacular way. When an individual goes through this incredible journey, this massive change in their life is rather confronting. It is cathartic, it is scary and at the same time exciting!

Here's the thing. When you dress an individual that has lost a bunch of weight over a short period of time, they have absolutely no wardrobe and their new body shape is something new to them. With the right styling, the contestants can look even slimmer than their new bodies. I had a contestant to make over and the results blew us both away.

Confidence was at an all time high, attitude was super positive and that meant a whole new outlook on life.

To wrap up this chapter, you can look slimmer if you dress with particular emphasis on the hems and finishes— the finer details matter. Be sure to look for symmetry and balance in each of your outfits. Contrast is king! Ultimately it's up to you and how you wish to be portrayed, however if you wish to look ten pounds lighter or to slim down your overall look, try the tips I've outlined on how to do this.

TAKEAWAYS

- Get to know your unique fit, color, and style.
- Check the mirror every time you leave home.
- Tailoring is essential.
- Contrast is king.

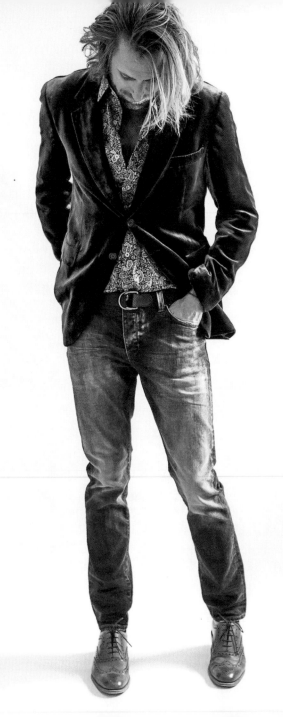

Chapter Sixteen

HOW TO DRESS FOR SEX APPEAL

We all want to look our very best and having sex appeal is part of it. Do you want to be more attractive, more sexy? A good place to start is to be thoughtful. Think about your date and the dress code that is appropriate for the venue where you are meeting.

For women to look sexy, it's pretty straight forward. Throw on a little black dress and some killer heels, some make up and boom! But how do gents dress to look sexy?

What's the male equivalent of the 'little black dress'? One thing is for sure, black is a very sexy color and that hasn't changed over the decades.

What to wear to dress for sex appeal

- *Black is the go-to sexy color.*
- *Fitted lines are the go to shape your body.*
- *Velvet or leather are the sexiest products to wear in jackets. However, try to avoid wearing trousers in these fabrications unless you're Jay Z.*
- *Last but not least, remember, every man looks good in a well-fitted tailored suit.*

Dress for the occasion. This shows respect. When you feel like you have achieved the right look for the environment, this in turn brings confidence.

A sexy look at your local bar could be the 'I haven't tried too hard' slightly disheveled look with a well-fitted pair of jeans, t-shirt and military or biker boot.

Your ensemble for a slick bar might be a well-cut suit and relaxed open neck shirt or knit and a pair of suede loafers.

Make sure you put some time into good grooming. This alone shows that you have taken some time and that you care about yourself. Check your shoes. Make sure they are clean and work well with your outfit.

Chivalry in a modern man is all too rare, so be the rare. Be punctual, it's attractive. But don't become impatient when your date is inevitably running late.

Whatever the situation, whether you are meeting at the local bar or a city night spot, confidence is key. Be authentic and that means looking like the guy that you are inside.

Don't be cocky or too full of yourself—that's very unattractive. The word authentic keeps coming up. There's nothing worse than being a fraud.

TAKEWAYS

- Good grooming will stand out so make the effort.
- Well-maintained shoes will be noticed and appreciated.
- Be chivalrous. It's genuine charm, it's being mindful, thoughtful and considerate.
- And the single sexiest thing a man can do, drum roll please ... show confidence. This will come from wearing an outfit you look and feel amazing in.

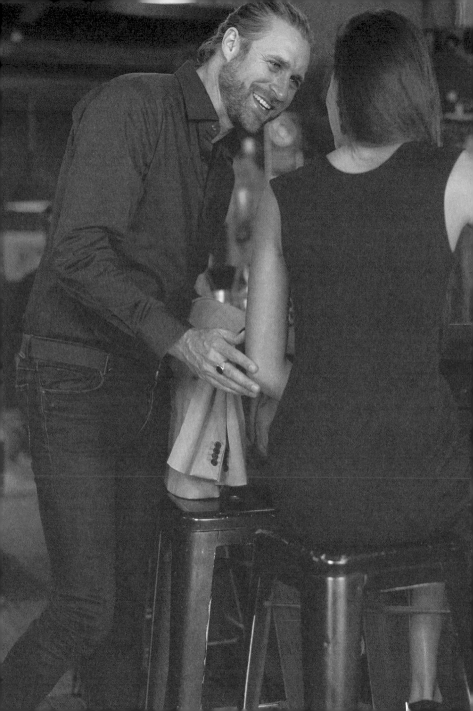

Chapter Seventeen

DATE NIGHT

You don't want to look over dressed or under dressed on date night. The first impression is imperative if you want to get to a second date.

You want your date's opinion of you to be closer to the authentic you so there is less explaining to do. Don't worry, your date will be making 50 assumptions about you. You may as well have them be good ones.

We pretty much fall into three basic dress codes for dating which I have called: the fancy restaurant outfit, the funky bar outfit and the blind date outfit.

Fear not gentlemen, here are my fail-safe tips for making a lasting first impression. Firstly, for any date situation, general grooming applies. Make sure you shower, shave (or trim), use deodorant, and splash on some cologne. And do your hair.

Now let's see what you can wear to impress on your date night.

FANCY RESTAURANT OUTFIT

Start with some dark denim trousers, tuck in your favorite dress shirt, throw on a matching belt, add lace-up shoes, and finish the look with a blazer (even if it's too hot to wear —you can take it off in the restaurant).

FUNKY BAR OUTFIT

This look calls for washed denim jeans, a plain well cut t-shirt, loafers, and to finish the look, add a blazer (or blazer unbuttoned over a shirt). If you're a waistcoat kind of guy, this would be a suitable option.

BLIND DATE OUTFIT

The perfect look starts with chinos, denim shirt untucked or a front tuck behind a canvas belt and casual boots.

Whatever the venue, it's important that you're confident in your look so you can relax and enjoy yourself.

Date night may be the start of something; a stepping stone to bigger and better things. Do yourself a favor, put in the effort to create a lasting positive first impression and it will pay off ten fold.

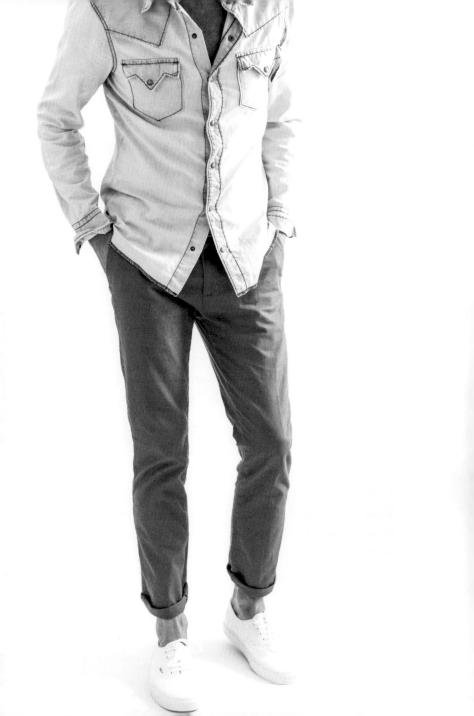

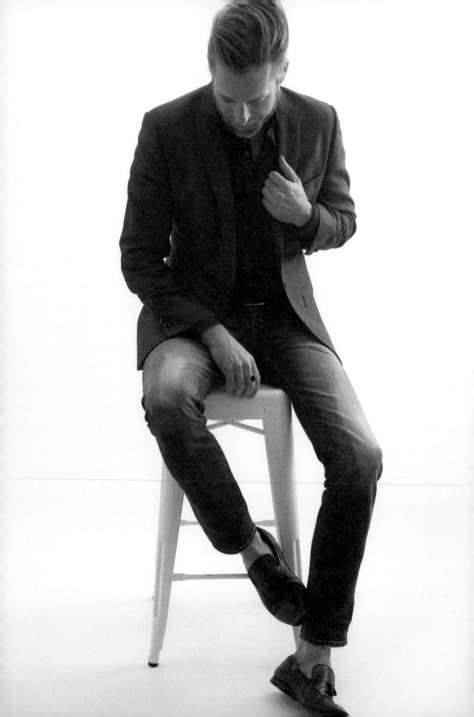

TAKEAWAYS

- Consider the venue when choosing your outfit.
- Consider your date when making your clothing choice.
- You can always dress down if you are over dressed—take off your jacket, loosen your tie.
- The first impression counts so be sure it's a good one.

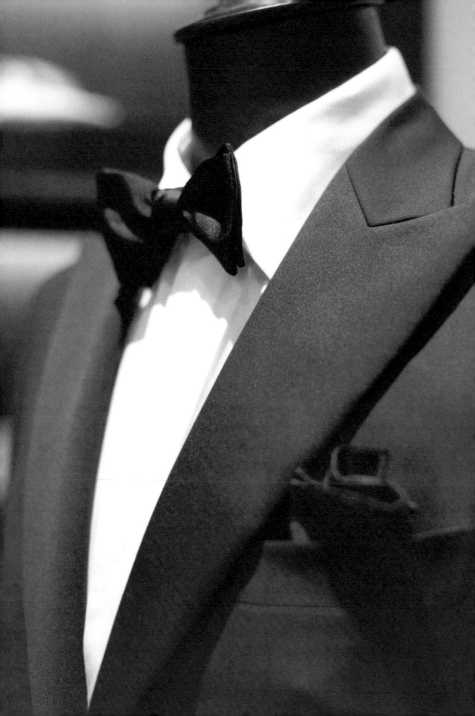

Chapter Eighteen

IT'S YOUR WEDDING DAY!

Grooms historically leave everything until the last minute. Too many times I have heard, "It will be alright on the night." Plenty of movies have captured the farce that happens between the buck's party and the wedding day. In movies it may be funny, in reality it is cringeworthy to watch unfold.

From white socks with a black tuxedo to completely mismatched suits (a no-no), wedding parties are a minefield of disasters just waiting to happen. I have had grooms stain shirts, rip jackets and pants on the morning of the wedding all to be sorted in time for the church bells.

Take the experience of Jeremy for instance. Jeremy had three groomsmen from interstate converging the day before the wedding to fit their suits. What could possibly go wrong? Two out of three well-fitted suits isn't bad, is it? Well no, not really, the wedding day calls for 100 percent accuracy. Suit three is not fitting the groomsmen anywhere, anytime soon. Who measured this thing up? The man needs spectacles! We needed to get this sorted ASAP.

Jeremy's groomsman, Isaac is not an 'off the peg' fit. Jeremy needed to purchase and tailor a new suit in two and a half hours. As Jeremy is a mate, I called my local tailor and asked him if he could take a rush job in the next hour. He obliged. We hit the shops like a hurricane and scooped up a suitable replacement in 30 minutes and then jetted to the tailor for pinning, cutting and sewing. This takes about 50 minutes. Clearly the only thing we can do is drink beer while we wait. Ok, let's check the fit. All good so we are soon en route to the hotel with about 15 minutes to spare. Talk about a close call!

What could have made things easier in the above scenario?

If you want to look your very best on your wedding day, be prepared. Have a plan (and backup plan) for each stage and element of the wedding. Put together a production schedule with your best man so you both know what's happening.

If you have groomsmen coming from elsewhere, having a tailor on standby (arranged in advance) would be an option. It could also have been good to have the groomsmen arrive earlier for a final fitting of all suits at least a few days prior to the wedding day.

It's super important to know what is available, how much

everything will cost and where you can get it. This enables eleventh hour decisions to be executed with precision and minimal fallout.

Weddings are the day you're meant to look your best. Even if it's your second go around, put some effort in. The photos are going to be around a long time. You had better look the part.

Everything needs to be turned up, not just to 10—turn it up to 11—your best look, your best grooming, your best energy.

Now I've scared you, let's take a closer look. The good news is there is a way to work this out. So let's get real about how to get this right.

STEPS FOR A HASSLE-FREE WEDDING DAY

When it comes to being a groom, tradition dictates that your style takes a backseat to the bride's. However, this doesn't mean your formal wear won't require thought. In fact, with all the planning you may forget to take care of your own style needs.

To help you out, below is a checklist with a timeline that will help keep you on track. Thanks to wedding expert and tailor to the stars, Wil Valor, for helping put together these 'steps to success'.

Three months out

About three months before the wedding, start by getting fitted for your suit—three months is the absolute minimum time to start.

Realistically, the sooner the better, this way there will

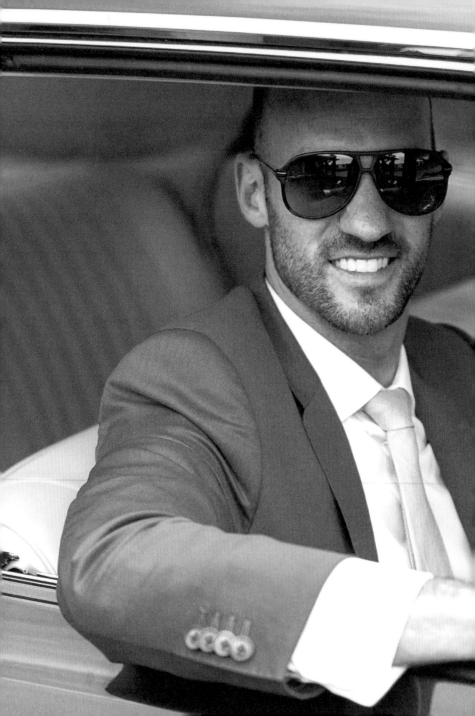

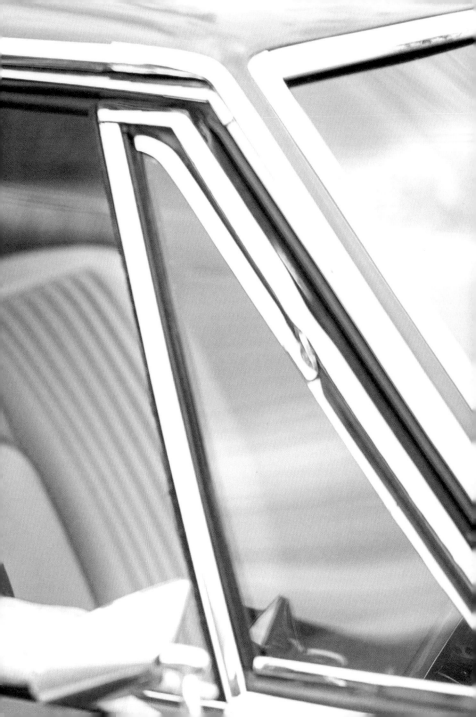

be no issues. You'll also want to allow plenty of time to get your groomsmen in for a fitting. Give them a due date that's a little sooner than you really need. Guys are notorious procrastinators when it comes to getting fitted for formal wear.

One month
It's back to your tailor to double check and make sure any alterations are perfect. Although a month out seems a little excessive, it will give you time to correct any mistakes or make up for any weight you've gained or lost since your initial fitting.

A week before
It's time to start working on some of the details. This is a good time to get a haircut. It will give you some time to have a little bit of growth but you won't have that 'new haircut' look. It's also a good time to do any other sort of personal grooming. Start cleaning up facial hair along with your new haircut. This is also a good time to look at the suit to see if it needs a final press.

The day before
Pay a visit to where you are dressing on the day of your wedding. Make sure you have all you need for the day. Double check to make sure you have your suit, shirt, tie, shoes, socks, vest, cuff links and any personal effects like razors, shaving cream, soap, hair products and toothbrush. Also remember the rings!

The big day

Hopefully by now you'll be on cruise control because you've thought ahead and prepared. Still there are things that must be done. Do your final grooming and get a good close shave. Also don't forget your deodorant; we tend to sweat during big moments. Check those rings one more time and then hand them to your best man.

The final step will probably be the biggest moment in your life. Since you know all the logistics are taken care of, you'll be able to take in the moment and enjoy your day.

TAKEAWAYS

- Allow extra time for every activity just to be safe.
- Create a working document you can share with your best man—this is your production schedule.
- Have a clear timetable.
- Keep a record of all pertinent phone numbers including emergency contacts such as your stylist, drivers, photographer, hotel and reception venue.

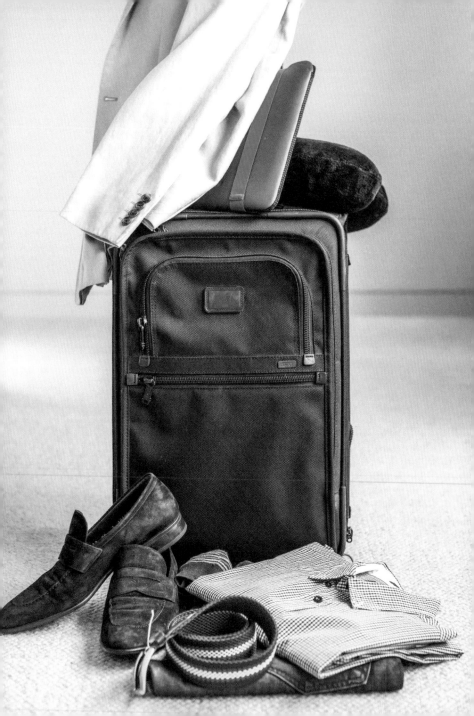

Chapter Nineteen

TRAVEL PACKING

Can you pack for a week away in an overnight bag? How do you pack for a month overseas?

Check your itinerary and the temperatures of where you will be going. Where will you be wearing your clothes? What will you be doing? What types of venues will you be going to? Will you be shopping for clothes?

I love to travel. I love other cultures and places. The inspiration of other cultures and people is intoxicating.

But I'm one of those guys who has never really loved some of the aspects of travel like checking in and checking out. Being tall, I don't love flights much either. However, efficiency is one of the things that I do love. I'm on a journey to enjoy the magic so streamlining the logistics is important. One way to do this is to pack lightly. This counts even more

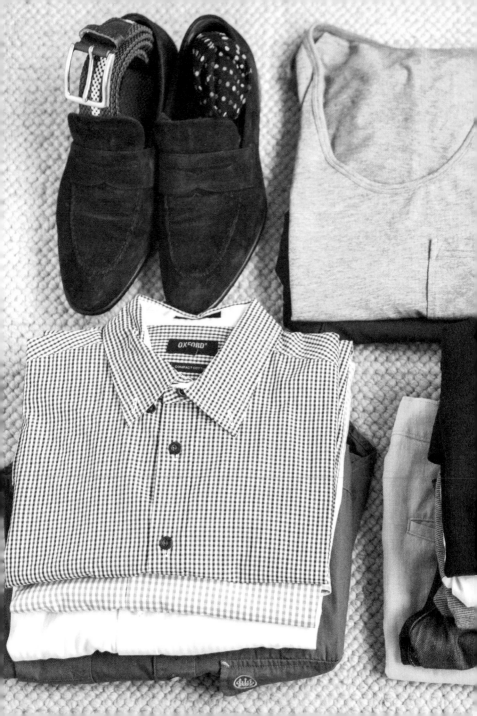

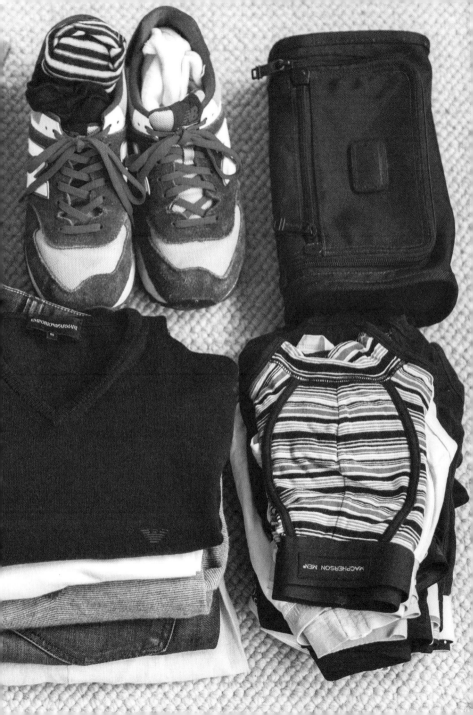

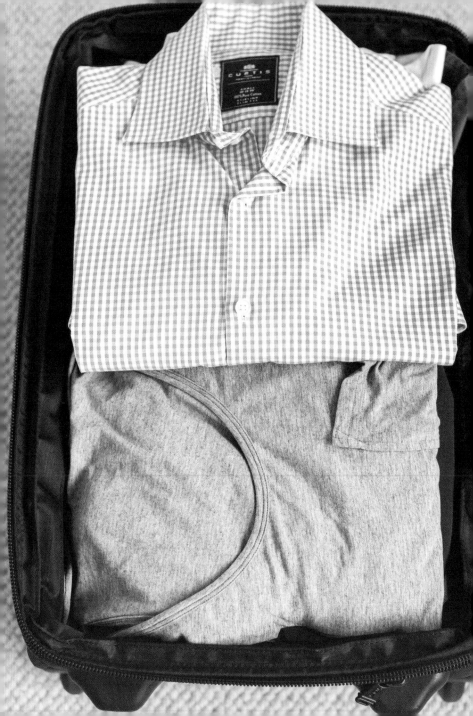

when I am going to be shopping on my trip. In this case, I'll pack even lighter so that I can collect some special pieces without needing to purchase another suitcase.

If I'm going away for anything from a two-day to a two-week trip, I pack a small overnight bag. If I'm going away for longer, I take a check-in bag and an overnight bag to carry on the plane.

It's important to have your everyday things accessible, such as toiletries and some leisure wear. Official documents and electronics should be in your carry-on luggage to keep them secure.

I'm not one of those guys who wants to constantly battle with an over-packed suitcase at every hotel I land at. Minimalism and organization are the keys to packing lightly.

A guide to minimalist packing

- *Make do with fewer things and use a cleaning service at your destination.*
- *Take the most versatile pieces to create the most combinations possible.*
- *Pack outfits that are stylish and functional.*
- *Be mindful of the weather where you are going.*
- *Make sure you have outfits for the occasions you will be attending.*

Most people only use 20 percent of their wardrobe that they pack so cull before you leave. Put all your gear together that you want to take, then reduce to a half. Do the same again until you have the very minimum that you will take.

Taking pressed shirts with you means they will require

pressing again, so I tend to pack shirts that don't wrinkle. Granted you don't want to be ironing while you're away. If you have shirts that need a press, ask the hotel to look after the ironing when you check in. Some hotels are moving to 'do your own' with irons and ironing boards in rooms.

If you are traveling to one of the fashion meccas such as London (best menswear shopping on the planet), Rome, Florence, Paris or New York, consider buying an extra bag and fill it up with locally-sourced, unique wardrobe pieces. I certainly wasn't planning to buy two vintage jackets on my last trip to Florence, but there was no way I wasn't going home without those gems.

My top tip for travel is to carry the heaviest coat or jacket on your arm to take it on board the plane. This will help to make sure your suitcase is not over the allowed weight. If you are carrying a suit bag, ask the air stewards to hang it for you.

TAKEAWAYS

- Minimalism is the key to successful travel packing, so take only what you need.
- Check your itinerary to see what events you need to dress for and pack accordingly.
- Use a cleaning service at your destination to minimize the amount of clothing you travel with.
- Buy an extra bag or suitcase if you spend up big.

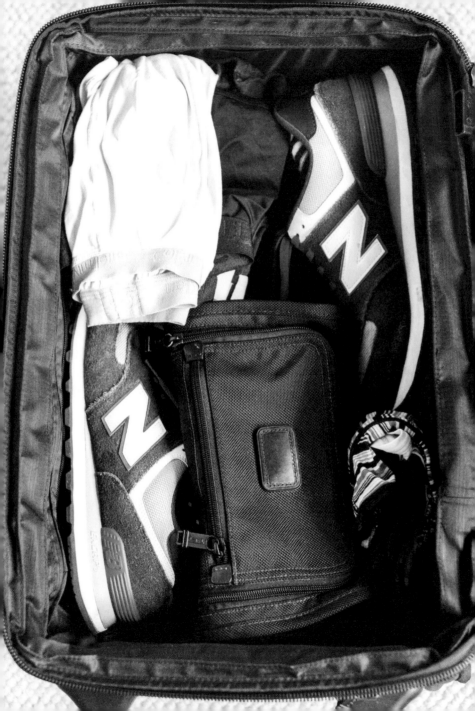

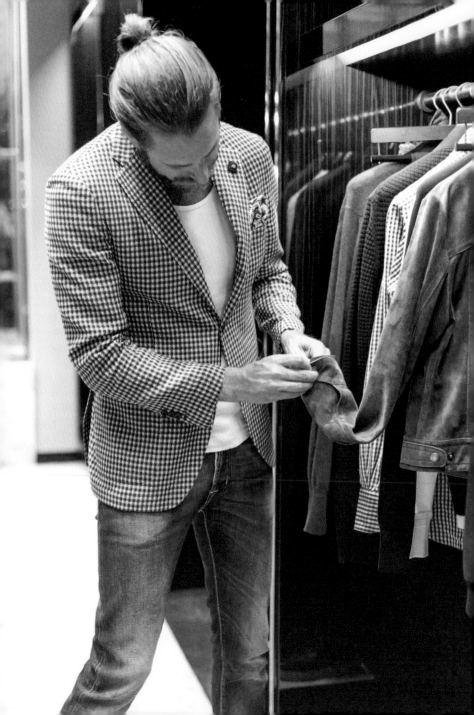

Chapter Twenty

SHOP LIKE A MAN ON A MISSION

Have you ever been dragged around the shops in perfect weather while you could be surfing, playing golf or watching paint dry? Shopping can be an absolute nightmare and a sure fire way to put pressure on friendships and relationships. Cue *Mission Impossible* theme music, slide into some comfortable shoes and prepare to cut through the transient retail sales staff random 'off the cuff' compliments, brave the hoards of happy shoppers and line up for a fitting room ... it's time to shop.

The first thing to do before you even hit the shops, is prepare.

Your shopping guide—before you start

- *Create a wish list of the pieces that are missing from your wardrobe.*
- *Source the wish list. Find the clothes online (and then in stores) and don't be distracted by things that appeal to you that are not on the list.*
- *Take a stylist or a friend who tells it to you straight. Lord knows the sales-driven compliments are rarely authentic. Ever been told you look great in something hideous or too tight? It is important to get sound advice.*
- *If you are in between sizes or the item appears too long or too short, look at tailoring that suits your body shape. A good tailor is your wardrobe's best friend. If you can develop a good rapport with a tailor, you'll get faster turn around times. And you're likely to get good quality workmanship.*
- *Don't buy something just because it is on sale; it is likely to be on sale for a reason.*
- *Don't compromise. If you do, most likely you'll never wear the piece or at best wear it once and never really feel it is right.*
- *I know this seems so simple, however, if you can't find the size in store in the color you like, ask for another color and if it fits, then ask the sales assistant to order one in for you in the right color.*
- *When you find a proactive diligent sales person, praise him/her and see what days the person is usually rostered to work. Call up prior to your visit to make certain this key person is available. A really diligent sales person may even prepare some looks prior to your*

arrival. Having someone reliable to assist you who has had experience with you in the past is a great person to have in your network.

SEASONAL TOP UPS

Once you have the basic wardrobe essentials, throw in some seasonal color and trend pieces to give your wardrobe a lift.

Each season there are new colors to choose from and every couple of seasons you will see new cuts or shapes as well. Top up as required.

TWO WORDS OF ADVICE

Just because a color is in fashion, it doesn't mean it will suit you. Drop crutch trousers may be in fashion, but it does not mean they suit you.

Shopping can be seen as, and has been called, an extreme sport. It is for me. I walk fast, talk fast, make fast decisions.

With the right supportive retail staff, we can make shopping happen about three to four times faster than you would on your own.

TAKEAWAYS

- Make a wish list and don't get distracted by sale items.
- Source online and then in stores.
- Take a stylist or friend who'll give you the truth.
- Don't compromise and buy something you don't really want or need.

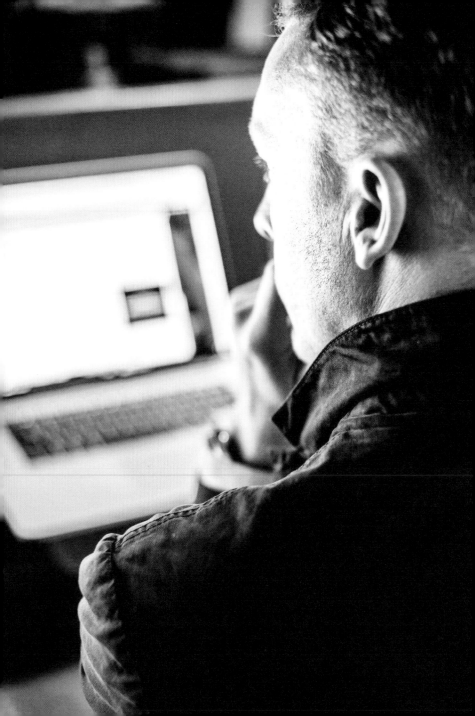

Chapter Twenty One

ONLINE SHOPPING

Online shopping is blowing up in a big way. The uptake in men's online shopping is growing at a fast rate, in fact, at the time this guide was printed, it was faster than the growth of women's online stores. But what are the pitfalls?

Why did it take us gents so long to embrace this shopping experience? How do you make the most of the deals that come up at sale time? How secure is it to shop on these websites? How do you make certain you have the right size? How do you ultimately avoid the returns process and make the purchase/sale a smooth, enjoyable even exciting experience?

Personally, I have had no trouble shopping online. Here's a couple of my experiences.

I always wanted a pair of white denim jeans, and lets be

fair, they are not readily available for sale at retail stores. One day cruising the 'Mr Porter' website. I spotted what looked like a pretty cool slim fit Acne brand white denim jeans. So, I check out the video and read up on the size guide and what size the model is wearing and I order a pair, considering that typically I take a size smaller so they fit better after the usual stretching.

The jeans arrived in days. I quickly tried them on and found I needed an extra inch in the waist. The website clearly stated the returns policy, so I sent them back and in no time had a replacement pair in the correct size.

Next up I started selecting things on my wish list and waited for them to come up on sale in my size. It is worth subscribing so that you don't miss out on sale alerts. When a couple of pieces hit my radar, I went ahead and ordered with a little more attention to the fit notes on the site. When this order arrived it kind of felt like Christmas as I had three new pieces and they all fitted perfectly. Awesome!

Another experience I had was with the shopping portal called 'Coggles' based in the UK. I spotted a lime green pair of slim cut, cropped chinos. They reminded me of a pair I had seen on my last trip to Paris so I checked out the specific fit and style notes and ordered them. These guys were pretty slow, so initially I was disappointed but here's the clincher!

This pair of trousers has never been available in 'real' stores where I live. I get asked about them and complimented on them every time I wear them. That's a win!

It does feel good, even a little special to have something no one in your area has. It's a little bit like the individuality of buying bespoke (see Chapter 10).

One of the drawbacks of online shopping for a lot of men is the return process. Even when buying from retail stores, it's just a massive pain in the butt to take things back for an exchange or refund. However, online returns policies are pretty straight forward for most labels most of the time. They're not as difficult as you may imagine, as the e-tailer needs to make the experience as user friendly as possible.

Ultimately, for anyone who dislikes shopping and is also time poor, online shopping is a revelation. It really won't hurt to dip your toe in the online shopping pool and check the temperature; you never know it could be the best thing since the goatee beard.

TAKEAWAYS

- Bookmark the sites you like.
- Subscribe to the e-newsletter for sale alerts.
- Select your favorites and put them on a wish list.
- Work out your correct size from the international size chart.
- Check the exchange rate.
- Check and follow the returns policy as some are only 14-day returns.
- Look for things that are not readily available at your local stores.

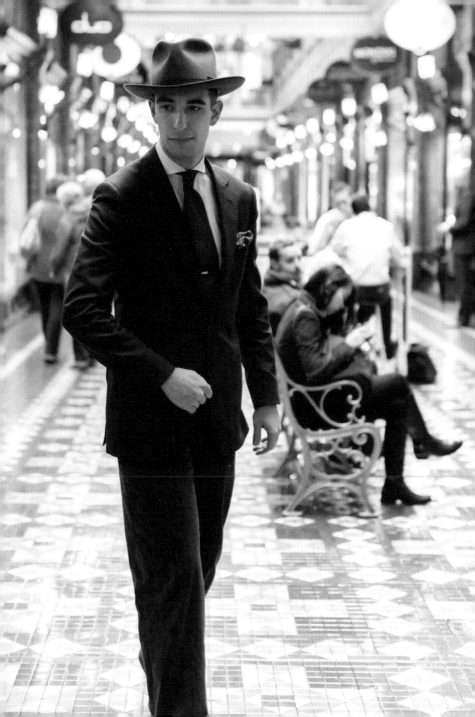

Chapter Twenty Two

INSPIRATION

How do you keep your creative juices flowing? We all get stuck in a style rut at times. We have all had that feeling that 'I have nothing to wear' and not being inspired by what we see in our wardrobes.

I find inspiration particularly when I travel whether at home or abroad. What people choose to wear in their particular environment, inspiration can be found by just walking down any street. It fascinates me and gives me ideas about color combination as well as layering.

You don't need to travel in order to be inspired with the amount of free information and images available on all forms of social media. From the comfort of your home or office you can be tantalised daily with stylish images from so many online sources.

For online inspiration, I recommend you create a central hub to access easily. One or two of the following sources will just click for you and when they do, pay this media a visit once a week to keep your looks fresh. Visit more often if you want more inspiration.

A guide to online inspriation

- *Tumblr, Facebook, Instagram and Pinterest as well as street style blogs are a great source of inspiration.*
- *Flipboard is an app for your phone or tablet that gives you a snapshot of all your feeds from multiple sources. This is a fantastic way to stay across what's happening without looking at every feed—like the day's news headlines personalised for you.*
- *TV shows and movies also give you styling ideas you may not find elsewhere. Think* Madmen, Boardwalk Empire, Game of Thrones *and others.*
- *There is no stigma attached to looking good as a modern man, so get your 'bromance' on and find a fellow style icon or two and try out some new looks.*
- *Compliments from men and/or women are always a good sign that you are on the right track.*

TAKEAWAY

- Keep an eye out for stylish locals when you travel.
- Look for inspiration online and create your own personal inspirational fashion and style news feed.
- Keep an eye out for gentlemen who are of a similar age group, build and coloring to emulate.

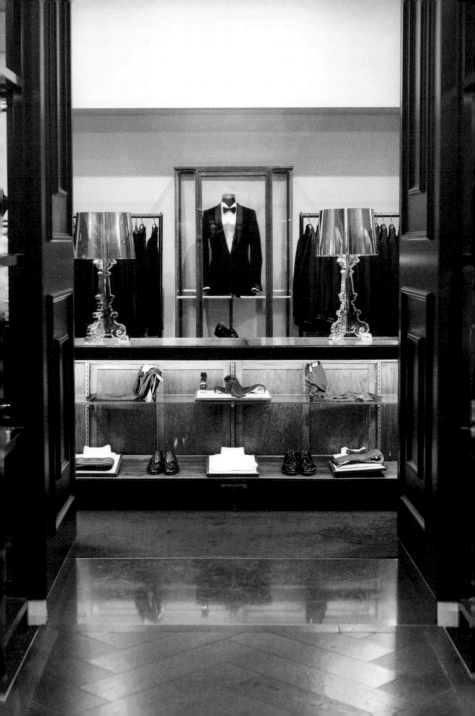

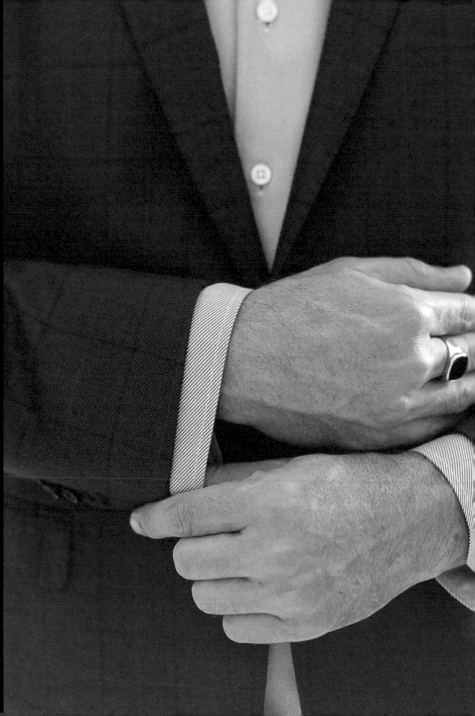

Chapter Twenty Three

STYLING TIPS

Every good book about style should have a summary of go-to tips that are a reminder of some of the most important elements of style.

Tip 1 Buy once, buy right.
With this philosophy you will save money, time, and keep you looking your best.
The 'buy once, buy right' philosophy means you get value for your money because what you buy will look good for a long time to come.

Tip 2 Denim needs to fit to look good.
Try jeans one size down as they always stretch. It will be a little uncomfortable at first, but it's worth persevering. If you can sit in them when you first try them that is a good sign. Make sure you have a neat even fit around the waist with no gaps (often the back of the waistband is gaping).

The waistline and thighs are the areas that stretch the most.

Selvedge or raw denim should be washed as little as possible. Try throwing them in the freezer inside a bag to take some of the smell out of them.

Tip 3 Buy loafers a half size down.
Slip on loafers will always stretch and once this happens your foot will just slip out rendering the shoes unwearable. Most important is that they feel firm but are not hurting you when you walk.

Tip 4 Dry clean your suits sparingly.
Pressing and cleaning fluids are volatile and spell the death of your favorite 'bag of fruit' if cleaned too often. Lightly sponge down minor spills and remember soda water is the best for mopping up red stains like sauce and wine. For a quick freshen up, hang your suit in the bathroom where the steam can easily flow through the garment

Tip 5 Follow the undo 2-button rule for wearing a shirt.
If you have just one button undone, it looks like you have just taken off your tie which can look a little stuffy. If you have three or more buttons undone, you can end up looking a little dated (so 1970s), or worse, you could look sleazy.

Tip 6 Choose the right collar to suit your build.
Pick a collar type to suit your neck shape. For gents with

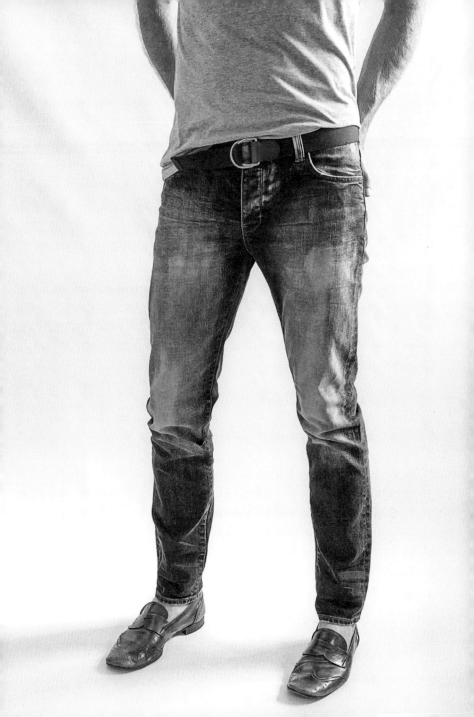

longer necks, try a higher or taller collar stand and if you have a shorter neck, a smaller stand will look more balanced.

Tip 7 Leave the last button (or bottom button) on all jackets and coats undone.

The last button is just for aesthetics. If you do it up, it will change the line of the jacket and it is not as flattering as it is if left undone.

Tip 8 Tie your knots (for ties) to suit the collar size of the shirt.

Large collars suit large knots but can also take a medium knot. However, a small collar only looks balanced with a small knot for the tie.

Tip 9 Tailoring will give you a perfect fit.

Tailoring is essential as nobody has a body that will fit perfectly for 'off the peg' apparel—this is why tailoring is best. The most common issue is sleeve length and the sleeves are usually too long.

Tip 10 Grooming is essential whatever your age.

You do not want the hairs growing out of your nose to spoil your style which it will. Grooming over 30? Hair growing out of every orifice? The solution is to wax, clip or laser—whatever you need to do to avoid embarrassment.

Tip 11 Wear fragrances that work for you.

Do wear deodorant (after bathing) and wear a fragrance

that works for your body scent.

The golden rule with fragrance is that if you can smell it in a strong way on your person, then it is going to be even stronger for your audience. Try a little on the neck and wrists and leave it at that. If you bath in it, that is down right sleazy.

Tip 12 Dress to the season.
No white trainers in winter, no boots in summer. Simple!

Tip 13 Untuck shirts when wearing trainers.
If you have your shirt tucked in, you will attain the full nerd effect. Not what you want. You want a casual look so untuck.

Tip 14 When to tuck in shirts.
Woven shirts can be tucked with smart shoes, however if the shoes are smart casual, this allows the option to go tucked or untucked. My tip here is if you are going to go untucked be sure to have your shirt hem no longer than your bum crease.

Tip 15 Belt up.
Belts don't have to match trousers for casual occasions. Try a canvas belt that coordinates with your jeans or trousers. However if you are wearing smart or dress shoes like a derby or brogue, you can match the belt with shoe color. Plate belts are for Batman. Just say no and buy a regular buckle—bigger for denim and smaller for trousers.

Tip 16 Coordinate a pocket square.
Pocket squares are super versatile but don't match them with your suit. Coordinate by matching to the tie, shirt or shoe color.

Tip 17 Check your trouser hemline.
Hemlines have come up in recent years however if you are running a shorter or cropped finish on your hems, the trouser should be tapered. Wide short hems are all wrong. Rolled chinos tapered finish pinch and roll is the way to go for relaxed casual looks.

Tip 18 Men's jewelry, do you or don't you?
Jewellery is often a contentious issue. If you remember to keep it masculine. Club rings or family rings often have a story so they work for this reason. Vintage can look good too. I personally don't love facial jewelry, however I do see its place in the music industry. Keep it masculine, keep it simple. If you think it's feminine then it probably is. Your choice in jewelry really tells a lot about a man, so make certain it's the story you wish to convey.

Tip 19 To man bag or not.
Controversial a few years ago, now you see them everywhere. Go for a bag that can carry what you need be wary of oversized bags; these simply look wrong. Check out your local markets for a vintage leather bag.

Tip 20 For color, contrast is king.
Make sure your contrasting colors don't clash and then go for it. Monochrome is great with an accent of color from accessories like shoes or a bag.

Tip 21 Don't sweat the smalls.
Socks and jocks—you can't have too many. Get them during the sales seasons. Cull the tatty ones.

Tip 22 How to offset a hangover.
A fresh white shirt and clean shave can cloak a hangover. Any facial hair on the cheeks will darken already tired eyes. White looks fresh and clean and most skin types will look brighter against white.

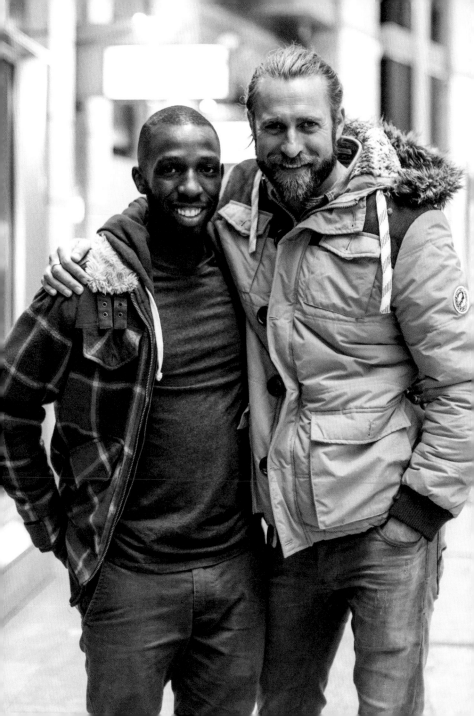

Chapter Twenty Four

INTERVIEWS

In the chapter on inspiration, I mention getting ideas from other gentlemen who are of similar age, size and coloring and whose dress sense you admire.

In this chapter, meet men from their twenties up, all with their own unique sense of style. They tell us how they developed their style, who and what inspires them and even divulge some of their more 'cringeworthy' moments as they grew up.

Find out which fashion designers are in vogue at the moment and more.

I hope some of these gents help to inspire you.

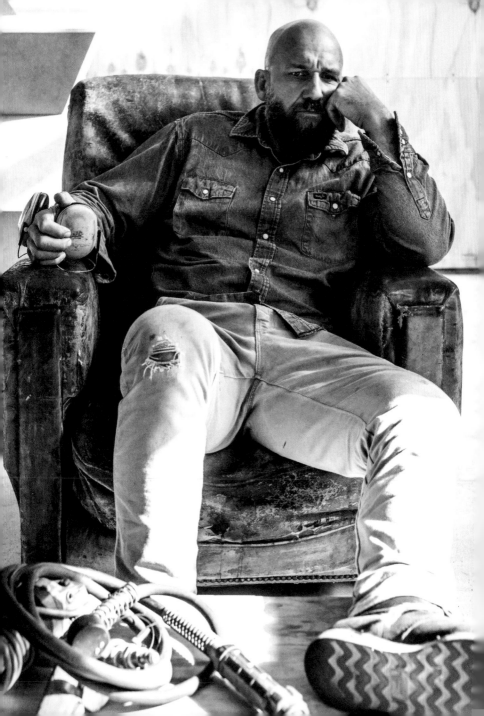

DION HORSTMANS

Dion Horstmans is a sculptor, husband and father of two daughters.

World famous, Horstmans' art can be seen around the globe with impressively large pieces donning high-rise building foyers and other scuptures shown in galleries, small boutiques and in private collections.

Salt water runs through his veins. That's why Dion loves living by the ocean and spends so much time on the beach.

Dion's 40-something frame is honed by a physical fitness routine that is a big part of Dion's life. However, riding around in his Pontiac is what he loves most when not sculpting or spending quality time with his family.

A lover of life, his personal style epitomizes modern masculinity.

What is your earliest recollection of dressing stylishly?

Probably around 11 years old. I'd saved up for a killer 'ocean pacific' (op) silk shirt. It had this huge tiger prowling through a bamboo jungle as the graphics—it was sick. Fast forward to my early years at high school; tapered school pants and pointy shoes, then skin tight black jeans, 14-hole DMs, braces and a collarless gray school shirt. Yup, I got sent home. I went back with a hair cut—a number two buzz cut. Got suspended for that one.

What/who influences your personal style?

I'd like to think I have my own style, but like every one, I'm influenced by what's going on around me. We're

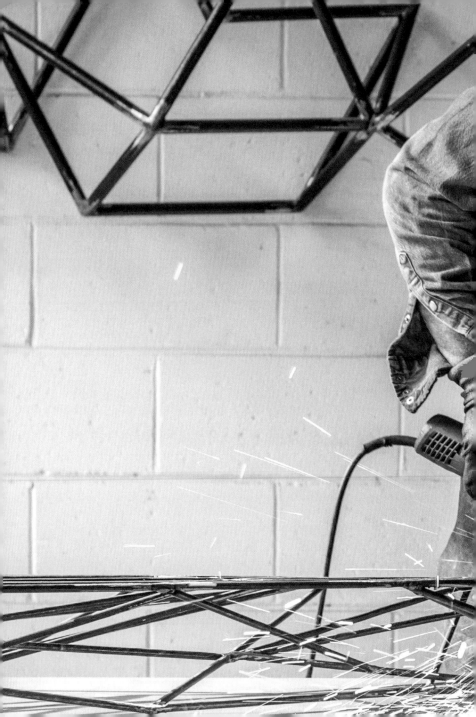

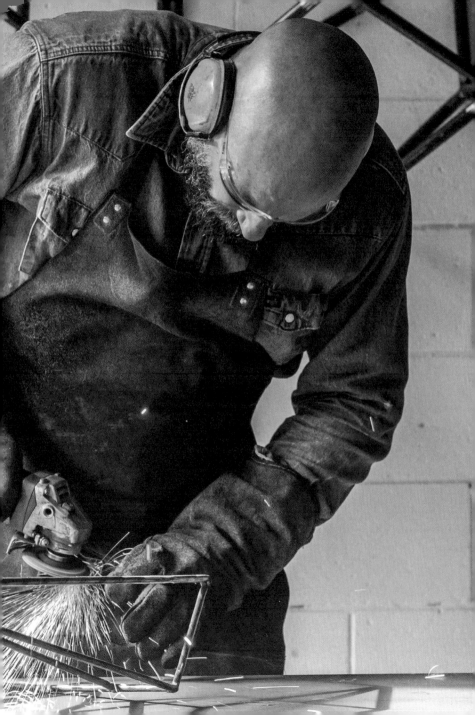

constantly bombarded with images. Subconsciously, I pull from everywhere. I'm a visual creature as we all are. I like simple lines. I like practical clothes. I don't think I've really changed much over the last 20 years. I love a pair of lace-up leather shoes, my boots, trainers. My wardrobe would be 70 percent Jac+Jack. I feel very comfortable in their shirts and knits.

I have two tailor-made suits from Zink and Sons, and a bunch of tailored shirts. I wear jeans or shorts.

Because I spend a lot of time at work, I'm in shorts most of the year, long sleeve denim shirts, a leather apron, and all the protective gear you need to work with burning hot metal—it's hot. If I were to think of fashion icons, I'd say Steve McQueen, Tom Ford, James Bond.

What style advice would you give?

Keep it simple. Be comfortable and confident in what you're wearing. Don't wear crocs unless you're a gardener, a chef or a young kid who has no choice because ya' parents bought them for you and you know no better. No ugg boots.

What's your favorite wardrobe piece?

Ooohhh, now that's a hard one. Off the bat, my two pairs of custom-made RM Williams boots. They're both buckle-up boots; one pair in brown leather, the other in a sand-colored suede. Secondly, my denim jacket. I've had it for over twenty years—a classic Diesel denim.

Favorite designer?

Hmmm, can't go past Tom Ford; ya' gotta love him. Hard to really choose one designer, our lives are full of beautifully-designed fashion and objects.

What's on your wish list?

A pair of black leather hipster jeans. I had a pair in the 90s, loved them. A black leather shirt, a pair of blue suede Gucci horse-buckle loafers and maybe a dinner suit.

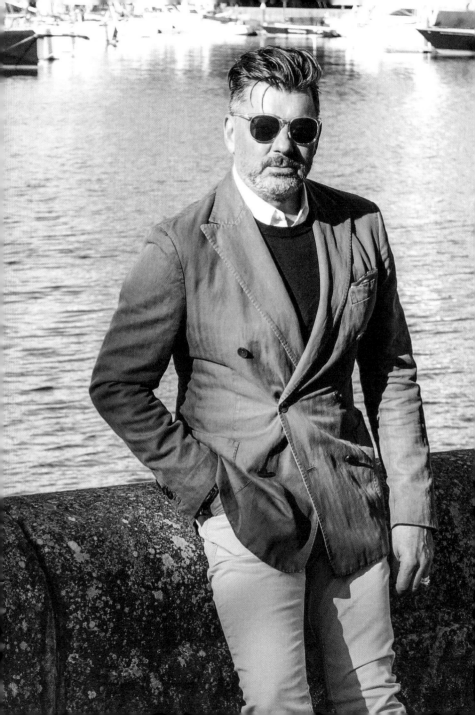

ALEX ZABOTTO-BENTLEY

Alex Zabotto-Bentley (aka AZB), former fashion editor, menswear designer and now event creator extraordinaire, is the owner of AZB creative, an event creation agency with a penchant for the flamboyant. AZBs multi award winning work can be seen all around the world in hotels and bars and at big fashion and lifestyle events.

AZB's Italian heritage is evident in his personal style and the uber creative events he and his team create.

With his background in fashion, AZB has a penchant for tailored garments, vintage design accessories and great footwear.

What is your earliest recollection of dressing stylishly?

I was very lucky growing up. My father was MC at the iconic San Remo Ballroom in Melbourne, Victoria in the 70s so he did all the big weddings for the Italian community and hosted dinner dances every Saturday; all in his perfectly tailored tuxedos. He was quite a role model. But my own style moment hit around age 16, when I got into New Wave. Those stylish groups like ABC (remember 'Poison Arrow' from their album, The Lexicon of Love?*), Echo and the Bunnymen, and Roxy Music.*

It was all about a dressed-up look—we were thrifting for 1950s suits, mixing in a little Rockabilly. Of course, I raided my dad's wardrobe for amazing tuxedo jackets; not just classic black, but deep burgundy brocade with black satin shawl lapels and creamy white with white silk lapels. I paired those with classic dress shirts and bow ties, baggy and re-tailored men's pants (with a seam down the back of the calf to make it extra tight). I nailed that look. I was young gun with such an attitude and an 11.00pm curfew. Rats!

Any cringeworthy childhood dress ups?
Growing up, I was a big fan of color mixing and matching and I became obsessed with finding just the right brown to go with the right green tee; I was a child of late 70s, remember. I recall seeing an album cover at an aunt's house; it was probably Slade or The Sweet or some glam band, and they were wearing head-to-toe denim—denim suits, no less. So, about a week later we were going to a family birthday and ma said she would buy my brother and I a new outfit each.

My bro was easy to please: a shirt from Merivale and Mr John and thick whale cords in mission brown. Done. However, I wanted that denim two-piece suit from the album cover. We made a pilgrimage to Myer and searched everywhere; kids, men's, designer, and then in young ladies (gulp),

I finally found a cropped denim jacket. Not quite a tailored mens suit jacket, but it was denim. I paired it with awesome super wide flared denim pants. I felt it wasn't quite right but it was a denim outfit, curated by me and procured by my ma. Perfect.

I wore the outfit with just a hint of cringe. It was definitely very Ted Mulray, with a David Bowie/Tina Arena slant. All went swimmingly until my godmother's sister arrived wearing the same outfit. But I wore it better!

What's the most powerful thing your dad taught you?

To always be a gentleman and to always care about the details. Being a gentleman: always introduce people, open the door for mostly everyone, be very polite and treat everyone with respect.

When it comes to personal style, it's about being elegant, regardless of whether you are in your Saturday hanging out clothes or your Sunday best. I always care about the details. An entire outfit can be ruined if the tie is not perfectly knotted.

What/who influences your personal style?

My personal style is a fusion of my present self and where I've been and my classic, slightly conservative Italian heritage. Growing up, I was a fashion renegade, smashing boundaries and reinterpreting trends with a keen, researched eye. I always needed to know the story behind a look and then I wanted to deconstruct it. Now I think I've found my natural rhythm. I hunt for brands and designers that follow their own mission, from Martin Margiela and Comme des Garçons, through to beautifully tailored brands like Tom Ford and Alessandro Dell'Aqua that are about the cloth and drape, the simplicity and the classic.

What style advice would you give?

Be aware of you, and put your personal stamp on what is around. You can't just copy a look you've seen in a magazine; style is not fashion and never should be. Style is the innate way in which someone sees garments and color and shape, then puts it all together to suit their own personality. It's important to find your own signature. But then again, clothing is just one small element of style.

What's your favorite wardrobe piece?

I have to choose? Impossible! That's like picking a favorite child. Well, if pushed, I'd say my Acne jeans, my Nike Air Max 90s Limited edition trainers, to-die-for Pal Zileri double-breasted blazers in an amazing eight-way stretch wool in washed navy and of course a serious shoe, Bottega Veneta hand-woven loafers. See, I told you I couldn't just pick one thing.

Favorite designer?

I have always loved the work of Cristóbal Balenciaga, obviously not for me to wear, but as an aesthete. I love the purity of his dialogue: the lines, incredible structure, his command of pattern making and his genius way with fabric. He responded to fabric like an interpreter; he created a whole new language of form and flow.

In terms of menswear I just love Martin Margiela. You wear his clothes; they don't wear you. He's a master of form and pattern, but with such subtlety and boundless imagination; a true master.

What's on your wish list?

Outfit: *a complete bespoke suit from Savile Row.*
Shoe: *Yves Saint Laurent fringed suede hi tops in Navaho brown.*
Watch: *gold Rolex President with original green face.*

Place: The island of Flores in Indonesia to build my massive Italianate dream villa.
Car: I'm on the hunt for a Porsche 911S 1974, original body, slightly modified.

What do you do when you run out of ideas; do you run out of creative energy?

Is this question for somebody else? I don't understand! My friends would tell you I am the fountain of ideas! I love the challenge of pulling apart concepts and repacking them and then pulling them apart etc etc. I won't run out of ideas until my brain gives up. There are always a million ideas buzzing around; the trick is how you interpret them and which ones you actualize and imbue with energy.

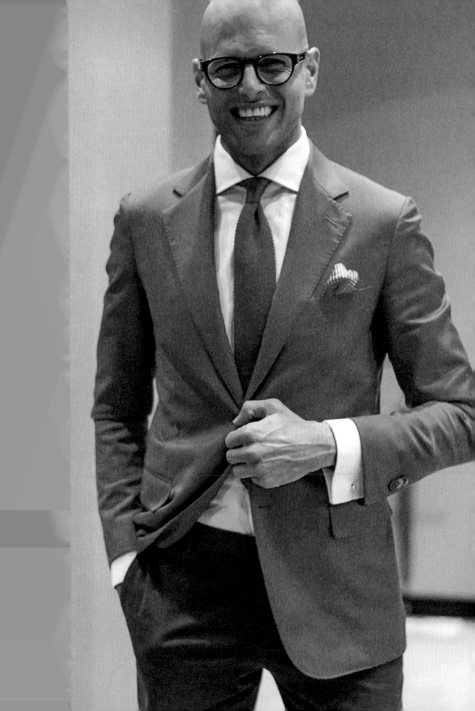

LUCA BRONZINO

Italian born, 30-something Luca Bronzino is a retail menswear manager in an exclusive luxury menswear store who loves styling his clients.

Influenced by his Italian heritage, bold colors and the finest details in accessories make up Luca's very polished look. Luca's signature Italian flair has helped him to become well known as a personal stylist.

Luca is a lover of the outdoors and enjoys getting to the beach in his downtime and taking in the sun and sights.

What is your earliest recollection of dressing stylishly?

From memory it was on my first day at high school. You see in Italy, we don't wear a uniform to school. My father had bought me a navy blazer for my first day of school. So I put together something that I thought was cool. I was wearing ripped jeans in a light color rolled up with a pair of white sneakers, fitted white shirt and tailored double-breasted navy blazer finishing it all up with a paisley pocket square in white and navy.

Any cringeworthy childhood dress ups?

A lot of denim, lots of white t-shirts. Nothing really loud, pretty casual, which is still my way today. Bomber jackets and lots of plain colors but the odd check shirt too. Nothing to cringeworthy after all.

What/who influences your personal style?

The city where I'm from, Pescara, which is a beautiful town right on the beach, where the weather is always beautiful. An incredible sandy coast from where you can admire the powerful color of the sky and where the sun reflects into the sea.

I get inspiration from magazines and just what people are wearing. From this, I get my passion for the light-weight fabrics and favorite colors, which are navy, white, lilac and beige which are all colors that you mostly wear in summer.

What style advice would you give?

Do not play hard with color combinations, and printed clothes. I play it pretty safe. Wear plain colors, and add prints with shirts and pocket squares that can add vibrance to your outfit. Ultimately look at where you wear your clothes, and choose styles that suit you.

What's your favorite wardrobe piece?

My three-piece PaL Zileri super-fitted plain navy suit. Soft shoulders natural line hand stitched. The waistcoat is double breasted and the cut is very slim and fits me perfectly.

What do you do when you run out of ideas?

I usually open a fashion magazine, and go through all of the beautiful images coming from the next season arriving from the best fashion photographers around the world. Also I like to watch the videos online of the fashion shows; the runway shows from Europe really inspire me.

Favorite designer?

My favorite designer is Tom Ford. I have admired him since he was working for Gucci. I will wear most of the clothes he makes.

What's on your wish list?

A super classic Prince of Wales double-breasted checked suit; double monk strap brown leather shoes; a black leather tote bag.

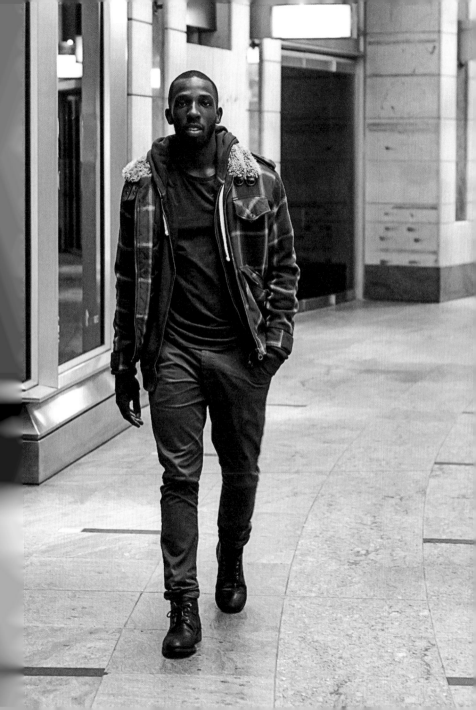

WILL NHONGO

Still in his 20s, Will is a part-time actor and financial markets tutor and researcher who has shared the screen with the likes of the popular Hollywood star, Hugh Jackman. As a keen sprinter, Will also trains and coaches young track and field athletes.

Flamboyant and outgoing, Will wears his personality literally on his sleeve with bold colors and clashing prints and textures. From beach apparel to elegant suiting, Will has an irreverent personal style always presenting himself in a positive, creative light.

What's your first memory of dressing in what you thought was really cool?
That would definitely be Sunday Mass. I would go to church, shoes were shined, the little suit was put on, crisp white shirt.

How far back?
That's like five years old. Obviously, my brother and I were matching, so that our mother could pick us out of the crowd. Same ties, same shirts, same shoes. I felt that was pretty stylish.

When did you start dressing yourself?
I started dressing myself in teens. The first time I tried to dress stylishly was definitely my school formal. And there is a picture of a baggy cream suite with a burgundy shirt and a cream tie, and some classic school shoe in dark brown. That was the height of metrosexuality at that time.

What did you learn from that?

Going to uni I learnt that you don't have to have the baggiest pants out and not to be scared of wearing something a bit more fitted. Even though at the time I was about 60 kilos.

What are your favorite colors that you wear?

I am a pretty colorful character. I prefer the brighter colors. Reds, greens, yellows, bright blues are my kind of palette. The bolder the better for me. With my skin tone as much as I would like to wear the charcoals and the blacks, they kinda' don't fit. White is also a bit too stark for me.

You grew up not having your old man. Was there another man in your life that influenced you?

Yes. My granddad. He was an absolute fixture in my life until he sadly passed away. He was the son of a man who walked from the southern tip of South Africa to Zimbabwe to find a better place. He had the deepest voice I ever heard. His voice sounded like a rumbling thunder. He always knew what needed to be said. He was a man with eight children on a farm and myself and even my mom never heard him raising his voice.

What impact did that have on you?

He was a very old school Englishman. He only wore tailored clothing and always wore a hat. That was because of the time when he grew up. He was a school teacher and very elegant.

So what's one thing that stood out that he taught you?

Grace. His infinite patience is something that I still wish I could get.

Tell me about your personal style.

I got very caught up when I was younger. If I could get my hand on any accessories, I was putting them on. So now it's just very simple, classic style jeans and t-shirt say a lot more than wearing mascots, 50 bracers, 10 rings, necklaces, sunnies and everything. It's just how I like to be.

How would you define your personal style?

It's just very simple. As I said, it's all about the classic casual style—jeans and t-shirts.

Can you explain further?

I'm not a minimalist, but I like 'natural'. I love the relaxed casual look. If I could get a look down to its simplest form, I do it.

When you are stuck, you have nothing left in your wardrobe, what do you do to bring creativity back to life?

I tap into my friends. I just call up some of my older mates who have all this knowledge of what is timeless and what is classic. They also know what's new and what's going be good next season; what colors I should be looking at.

How does technology affect how you consume fashion?

It's made it much easier. It was so difficult to find a way to make fashion work; it's about body shape, skin tone, personality. Before it was so difficult. But it changed with the advent of the Internet with its blogs, idealism and services. The trunk club in the US, is a good example. You can have a personal stylist who will help you to figure out solutions.

People can stumble across your blog and if you have half an hour to go through it, you can find a way to build a timeless wardrobe that is going to be stylish. So technology has opened things up for everyone wherever you live.

What about Instagram?

Instagram is huge as well. It makes it so much easier for me to find someone who is a style icon. To find out what that guy is doing right now, what is he looking at, what is he thinking about. That's how you get stuff that is good for you. Now you have democratic access.

What's on your wish list?

Tailored suit, hand-made shoes. My own custom luggage, that's something that not many people have. The crispest casual Alexander McQueen—I would have the sneakers and the jogging pants and the shorts. I would have everything from Alexander McQueen. It's so elegant. He's definitely my favorite designer.

Anything else you wish to add?

I think it's about self-confidence, love, humility and drive. The modern man can acknowledge desires to dominate. That's not necessarily a bad thing, however you need to be able to channel emotions in a way that enrich and unify those around you, especially those who you care about and love. If you can do that, that's the modern man for me.

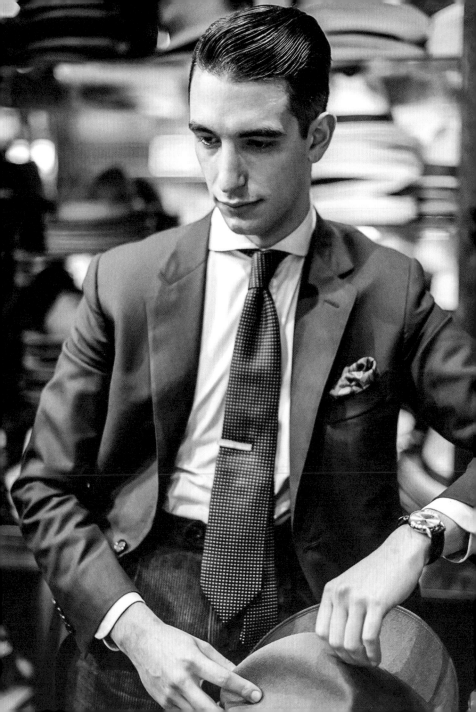

PETER HILL

Peter stands out in a crowd due to his stature and that he's nearly always seen wearing one hat or another. It may be why his personal style has been captured by many street style bloggers.

Modern vintage styling and vintage watches and accessories give 20-something Hill a unique look that always impresses.

Hill boasts a personal collection of over 70 hats—not surprising given that his day job is to style, fit and repair men's hats.

The music industry is well served by Peter's keen eye for headwear when styling his clients. Hill's modern look is undercut with beautiful tailoring in an ode to yesteryear.

When he's not styling his clients with the right headwear, Peter can be found playing his guitar.

What is your earliest recollection of dressing stylishly?

I think I remember pretty early on that I had bits and pieces that I would lean towards. There was this old tweed coat. I recall it didn't fit that well and it had a broken button, but I used to wear it with a t-shirt. I wore my first flat cap back then, cowboy boots and polished denim. The idea of structured clothing, I think, sort of fell in with me and I thought, this is cool. The coat thing was big for me. There were a few coats I picked up, like a vintage coat, a double-breasted, gold buttoned thing.

Any cringeworthy memories you wish to share?

I had red leather pants I had made up. Very Michael Jackson but that's what I wanted.

What inspired that?

Just listening to Motley Crue and heavy metal bands, that sort of thing. Originally, it was the biggest influence for me. I wanted big hair but I couldn't grow it long. It didn't work, but I looked like I was out of Guns N' Roses, at least I thought that's how I looked.

What did you learn from your dad or step dad?

The idea of buying quality. Buy things that last, don't invest too much in fashion as it turns over so quickly.

My dad would say things like, "This pair of boots? I've had for (xx) years and I'm going to polish 'em today." He looked after things and he always banged on about it which I think is 'A'. Those guys who are in their 50s and 60s now, they were definitely conscious of how they consumed.

What about your first memory of seeing something that impressed you?

I think that's the Aussie country prep. Like, you know, with the riding RM Williams boots, a kangaroo plait belt and moleskin jeans. That's actually really very Australian.

It's one of those things that doesn't get talked about much. But it's Australian country prep that you don't see so much now.

There's the older generation and their style is completely Australian. Any of those old farmers that you know. Anytime they came to town they dressed up. They wanted to look good. They weren't wearing their everyday work wear from the farm. They made special effort to present themselves in a dignified manner.

What style advice would you give?

I think taking the first steps is the most important thing. And making sure it's something you're comfortable with. For me, I have made a few bad decisions in clothing, you know, things that I didn't really wear, but I bought them because I wanted them and I felt that they reflected my style.

Learn what you like to wear. It should be a style that represents you.

Favorite wardrobe piece?

Definitely bespoke trousers at the moment, double pleats.

Would you like to design your own things?

Yes I'm picking up ideas, bits and pieces from where I see them and things like that.

What's inspiring your desire to design?

Film. You know, period films. I see stuff everywhere. But I love a lot of the old actors. Obviously Cary Grant, Marcello Mastroianni. Those guys wore what worked for them. Fred Astaire is a perfect example.

I wouldn't necessarily wear what Fred did, but he wore his clothes so well and looked the part because of that.

When you run out of ideas, what gets you going and going?

I tend to pull something random out of my wardrobe that I probably haven't worn for a while and try to wear it. It's sometimes really difficult to do it well but it's great when it comes together.

So you try to create something different when you do this?

Yes, like a pocket square that I probably never really thought about or pick a color that I never really thought would work for me. I'm not particularly great with some colors and I can experiment with them, where I can wear them and where I can't.

And again, going back to film sources and obviously the blogs I follow on the Internet—that sort of thing.

And what's your wish list?

Golden tassel loafers and cordovan. I think I need black for that future monochrome silver temple's look when I can start wearing gold. What else. I was in love with a beautiful loden coat like the old Venetian guys wear with the heavy box pleat, real long. Obviously move somewhere cold enough to wear it, just a few tailored pieces. I'm really craving texture at the moment. Donegal tweeds, that sort of thing. I need a new pair of jeans too, so trying to find the right pair.

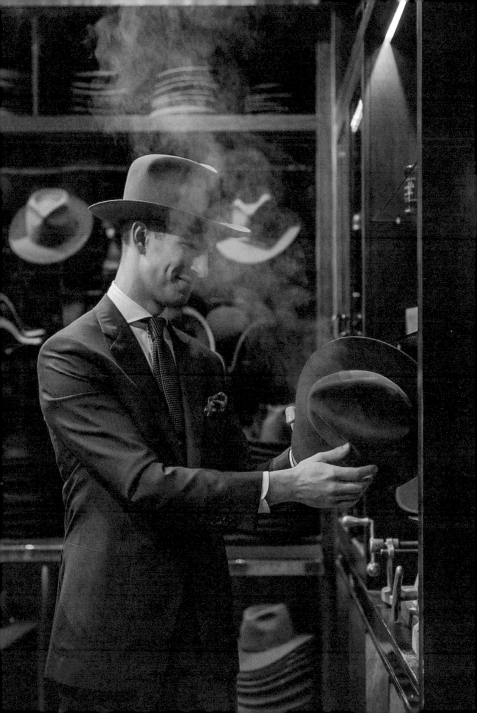

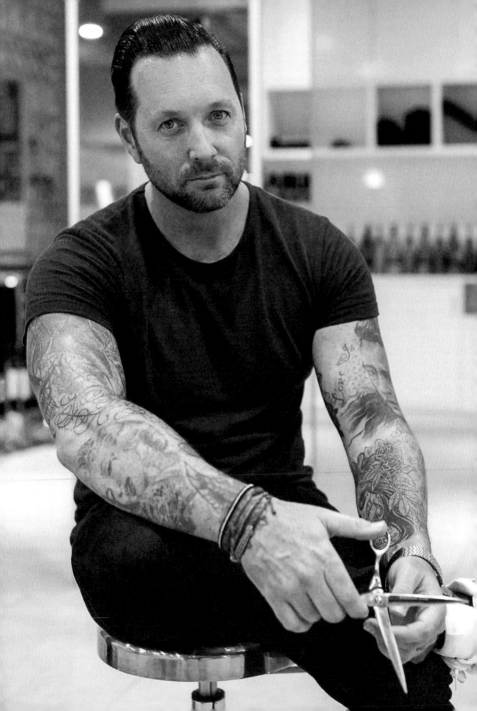

STEPHEN FOYLE

As Benjamin Button (aka Brad Pitt) looks younger as he gets older, so too does 40-something Stephen Foyle. Stephen who is GQ magazine's preferred hair stylist and is the creative director at Detail for Men, a hairdressing business that features actor, Guy Pearce on its website.

Stephen, who is passionate about empowering men to look and be their best self, travels to New York and other destinations for inspiration and recreation.

Sharpening up the edges to a classic 'bad boy' look, Stephen's skin art is as much a part of his personality as major influences from LA and Japanese fashion. Aside from an impressive sneaker collection, Stephen's clean-cut look is punctuated with neatly curated jewelry.

When was the first time you made an effort yourself and came up with an outfit?

I definitely had a sense of myself when I was 12 years old. I grew up on a farm and my sister said you don't even sound like us. And it wasn't because I'd heard someone else or I was copying someone else. I was influenced by that middle class space where I grew up.

That lack of conforming to any norm is really what I felt I needed to do. Essentially, there's a lot of pressure on young males to conform. If you allow it, it takes away a small grain of confidence. And I actually recognized that at a very young age.

I refused, from a young age, to conform to others' expectations. Not because I wanted to be different, it's because I wanted to be myself.

So what did your old man teach you?

Well, he actually taught me the most valuable thing and it wasn't intentional—what sort of shoes I wear to school or what sort of hairstyle I have can make a difference.

Being a male and seeing what has been done, evaluating the good and the bad and then moving forward and creating an action plan. Your grooming regime makes a strong statement. If you walk into a room in a suit (when that's the dress code), you create a different impression than if you walked in wearing a pair of board shorts.

How you present, changes the energy of a space; it changes the communication. Non-verbal communication can be more effective than words.

Any cringeworthy moments when you were dressed by your family or by yourself?

Yes, definitely. I think with any light there has to be darkness and I had some dark years. I have school photos of me with a slicked back, strange hairstyle a little bit pulled up through the fringe down my forehead color popped up. I suppose that could be classed as cringeworthy.

Every 10 years my style comes in and then I'm on top. And then I'm in the wilderness straight after that.

Given your early weird hairstyles, how did you become a hair stylist?

I started as an architectual student, and I planed to have my own practice. That was my dream. I suppose my personal style was always around.

Who influences you?

I've been influenced heavily by Johnny Cash. I think he was just an all-round, ultra-male dude. He's now permanently part of my fashion wardrobe.

Who is your favorite fashion designer?

Tom Ford and Hedi Slimane. Both for two different reasons. TF for the most masculine designs. He just captures what it means to be a male in his designs.

Hedi Slimane because he's contemporary and he's not bound by what's happened in the past. He looks forward to creating a whole new sense of masculinity for the younger generations, which is almost as important as celebrating the past. As a local designer, I like Brett Wilson because he's got a really smart way of cutting cloths. Very tailored. And, I think, guys at M.J. Bale—they've done some really strong stuff.

How does technology affect how you consume fashion?

I suppose, technology makes it easier for me to see options. But, as a consumer, everything I wear is tailored. Because you can never buy anything without it being tailored, whether it's a shirt or a jacket. Even if it's made by the best designer in the world, without it being tailored it depreciates dramatically. I suppose, the technology gives me variations of things that I might like, but I need to be tactile.

I need to see it on me and, more importantly, I need to customize it. So it only helps to facilitate what could be, not what I would buy.

Describe your job and how you influence modern masculinity.

My main role is to be a conduit between what men have, what men know, what they can be, and more importantly what they should be.

My main role really is to create happiness, so with that I use structural realities and not trend related realities. I don't listen to what's happening at the moment as a guiding fact. The males' facial features, their occupation, their height, their weight, their personality. But the absolute is their facial structure. Lean and tall, square shapes, jawlines. Using hair as a resource—that's my job.

What are your thoughts about make up on men?

Like anything, if the tool is used correctly, it's useful. It's not something that I personally would probably use. But for guys with scarification, pigmentation blemishes—if that helps them get to a level of confidence, then I think it's positive.

How has metrosexuality effected modern men?

I think the metrosexual movement was really useful, because things don't change in culture without controversy. Whatever that is.

It started a conversation with normal guys who actually deserve to have the same options available as women. Good grooming doesn't make you feminine. Good grooming actually makes you more masculine. That's what came out of the metrosexual movement and I think that was something really positive.

So you think grooming for men is important?

I think when it comes to grooming and men's fashion, it's always going to bring out a lot of emotions because people attach their own background, their own insecurity, their own lack of confidence to it.

They want to feel better about it by making other people feel the same way. That's changing. It's not going to happen instantly, but the modern man appreciates the fact that grooming is actually part of the uniform of success.

So feeling and looking good creates an attitude and that attitude shift creates money and success—whether that's about finding the right relationship or getting that promotion that you always wanted. Your confidence is now enhanced because of your aesthetic. Grooming is a tool and it's a powerful and essential one.

Why do you think you look younger now than say five years ago?

I think for me it is about having the confidence to walk into any situation and morph into my surroundings. But at the same time, display to people with elegance and sophistication that I'm quietly confident. And that itself speaks volumes.

What's on your wish list?

Pair of Churchill shoes—definitely brogues. I think they are classic.

I'd like to have a significant timepiece to pass onto my children. Patek Philippe primarily. I think that's a classic masculine piece. It uses that classic quality.

It's cool to have a look and it's cool for people to have a statement. That's great, that's personalisation. But men should really be groomed. They should have an overall sense of classicism. And that's masculinity. That's style.

I think I still have love for a gold submariner Rolex. And I think every man should have a trench.

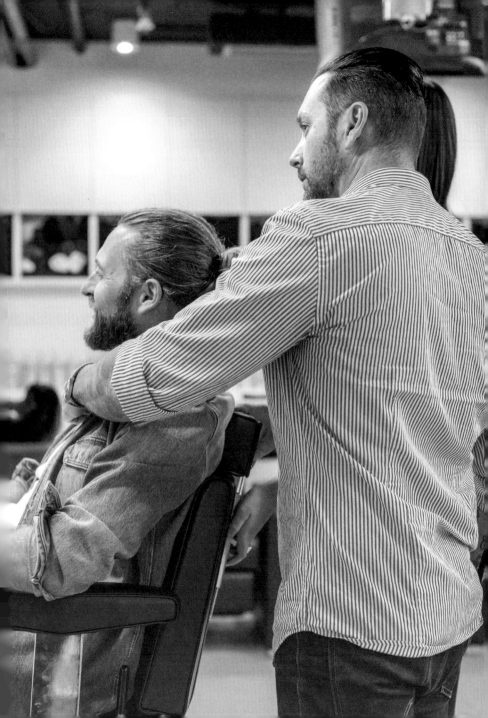

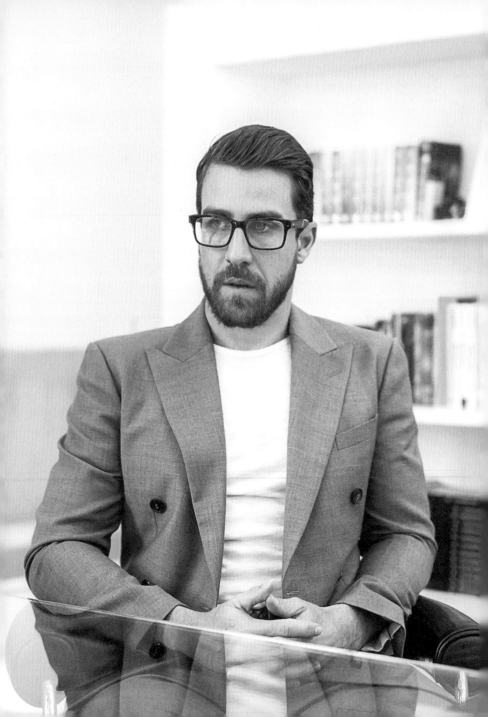

BRENT WILSON

Brent is a successful menswear designer. His brand specialises in affordable modern tailoring for men.

Brent's personal style includes tailoring with a relaxed twist such as wearing white sneakers with a double-breasted suit.

When Brent isn't designing, he loves to get physical to keep fit. However, his major passion is motor sports, so much so, that he spends most of his spare time racing motorbikes.

What's your earliest recollection of dressing up stylishly?

I don't go after all that's stylish, but my introduction into fashion was through surf wear. It was the early 90s; surf wear was massive. Even if you didn't surf, you still wore surf wear. That was definitely my first introduction.

I didn't really realize it before you brought that up. Big Australian surf wear labels like Rip Curl and Quiksilver, Mambo and Billabong, head to toe—that was me.

What would your favorite wardrobe piece be?

It depends. Top three pieces in a wardrobe would be pieces I can wear every day—depending on where I am, the surroundings and the weather.

What style advice would you like to share?

Get comfortable. Embrace your own individual personal stuff. Thinking about it, there is no right or wrong. If you want to wear something, wear it.

If you feel comfortable and that is you and your personality, go for it. You can't be governed by what I say or what anyone else says.

What about creative energy? How do you top that up?

Mostly through the little things. It might be something as simple as looking through Instagram. Sometimes that gives me ideas. Looking at what other people do pushes me to want to do better and be the best that I can be.

Going into stores, looking at what is happening on the streets, checking out luxury stores, looking at the presentations. What they are able to achieve is amazing.

It inspires me that maybe one day I can create a local brand as well. It's amazing, just walking down the street —sometimes the tiniest things give me inspiration and creativity.

How does technology affect how you consume fashion now?

The world is a small place now. Everything is in front of you. All the installations, ideas. You can see what's going on, you can see how the competitors are going.

It's very important that you don't lose track of who you are, where you are and where you're going. I think it's amazing.

Technology with the Internet and online stores gives the small brands— brands like my own and others a chance to advertise against big brands that have a lot of money behind them.

Favorite designer?

My favorite designers would have to be Tom Ford and Paul Smith. Different reasons for each. I like Paul Smith and how he created an incredible global brand. As a person he's not afraid to get his hands dirty. There's lots of articles where he's in a warehouse picking up boxes. So he's just a real people person.

Tom Ford? He's simply a very clever and creative individual.

What's on your wish list?

I'm not seeking fashion. I don't really seek it out. I can appreciate other people's clothing and design when I go to stores. That gives me inspiration for my own brand and pushes my creativity. But actually buying things—it's not really me.

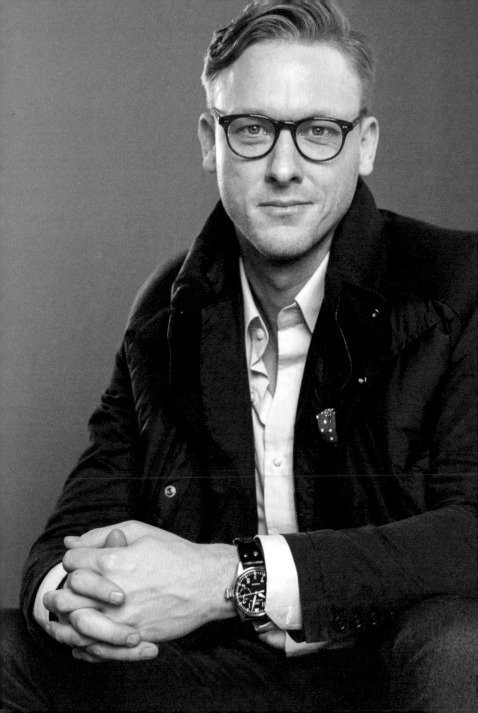

LUC WIESMAN

The founder of men's online publication D'Marge, Luc's knowledge of current and future fashion trends is second to none.

Over half a million visitors to his site each month means a lot of hard work for him and his team. Wiesman is addicted to training and works out as often as his gruelling travel itinerary allows.

Luc's ability to organize travel gear and to pack lightly means he can attend international fashion shows around the globe.

30-something Wiesman is mad for sneakers and boasts a huge collection, in fact, he rarely wears the same pair twice such is his passion. Luc has a sharp fashion edge and a dedication to self improvement.

What's your earliest recollection of dressing up?

I didn't come out of the womb dressed as a stylish guy. It took some time and some work to understand what style really was.

My parents traveled to the US for work quite often and this gave me access to the latest sneakers. I was aware of what was coming out so I would place my order and then I would be the first kid in school with the latest look.

It was through such experiences that I got a taste for nice things. I was always experimenting but it didn't always work.

Fashion was less of a concern when it came to my appearance because I had braces and that was my focus.

Any cringeworthy dress ups from your childhood you care to share?

My sister is ten years older than me, so I grew up with her giving me advice about what girls liked. This was the trade off for her dressing me up as a ballerina with a long wig and making me strike poses at her every whim. And I know you will ask—yes, there is photographic evidence.

What is the greatest lesson your dad taught you?

My dad is Dutch and cool. As a young man he had big curly hair and always wearing Ray-Ban aviators. His appreciation of watches and sunglasses and watches that were also cool has definitely rubbed off.

He also taught me to master an art, to be good at something. I tend to rush and he has slowed me down.

Who are the style icons who influence you personally?

Steve McQueen and Paul Newman are as good as it gets for me. But imagine if Steve McQueen could see kids taking selfies today? I think his advice would be, 'Don't be a showboat, be masculine and be a gent.' Chivalry from yesteryear is something that could be embraced now—but add Gosling crazy, stupid love.

Who is your favorite designer?

Designers come in and out of favor for me; my favorites change as I change. Right now South Korean, Woo Youngmi: his collection is tailored with a contemporary edge.

D&G fits me really well, so I can't go past the trousers in the collection at the moment. I have extra long arms so my shirts are bespoke. I also wear M2M suits.

How do you top up your creative energy?

It's travel for me and I travel quite a lot for work these days. After I got over my fear of flying, I really enjoy seeing what people are wearing all around the world.

European men dress so well and this inspires me. What they wear and how they create combinations is an art form. I would love to see men generally make this more of a way of their lives like the men do in Europe.

What's your favorite piece in your wardrobe?

My leather bomber jacket by Undercover a Japanese brand. It's a very expensive jacket that I picked up for 350 instead of 5k. I'm a fan of buying at sales. I also like pieces that are timeless like this leather jacket.

How do you spend your downtime?

Down time are you kidding? No seriously, my business (D'Marge) has taken all of my downtime over the past five years. Now I am exploring what downtime looks like.

I had a holiday with my family and it was just what I needed. It's easy to forget how important family is. Outside of this, I also enjoy exercise at the gym and outdoor activities.

What's on your wish list?

Burberry trench, as the weather requires this Gilet Monclur bright colored puffer jacket.

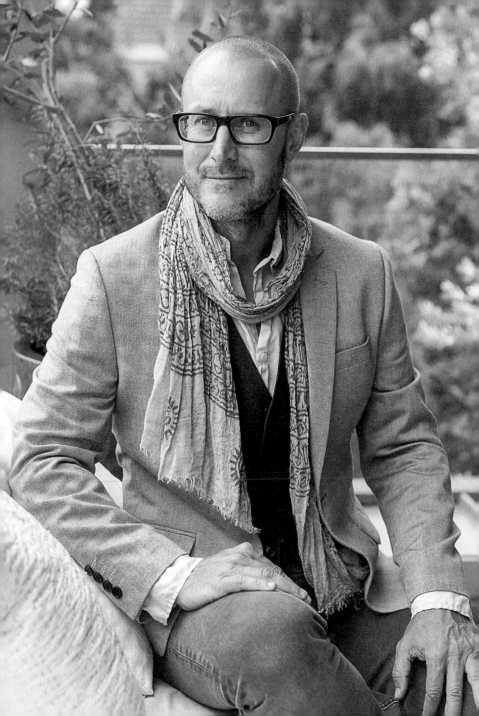

ANDREW HAMPSON

Andrew is a 40-something beach loving yoga instructor.

From popular advanced yoga classes to one-on-one celebrity clients, Andrew lives and breathes yoga. Check out 'Bad Yogi', his Instagram account for some lifestyle inspiration.

Andrew's personal style captures his coastal relaxed attitude to life. Embracing a considered mix of soft tailoring and grungy casual components, Andrew epitomizes the essence of modern masculinity through his chilled out, laid back manner.

So what is your earliest recollection of dressing up stylishly?

I guess for me, it's when I first earned some money. Funny enough there was a fashion store called 'Daily Male' near where I live. I used to go in there regularly and, kind of, basically spent all my money on buying items of clothing. Prior to that, certainly I was borrowing dad's shirts if I had something happening.

So you were a teenager at this point?

Yeah, 15 or 16. So initially I was borrowing Dads shirts and having something a bit more stylish to wear. Then as soon as I started work when I was 15, I had the money to spend as I wished.

Do you remember the first thing you bought? Or one of the first things that really took your eye?

The funny thing is I can remember a few items. I remember buying a pair of long yellow trousers that, at the time, to me, were very stylish. I do remember yellow trousers with a pink shirt and a gray thin tie. I recall that, somehow at the time I have no doubt that it actually looked ok. And I don't think it would have looked good for long though. But at the time it was alright.

And any cringeworthy moments from when you were a child and you had to be dressed up in anything?

When you get to reflect back 20 years, almost everything 20 years ago is cringeworthy.

I had this recollection of these shorts that went down below my knees and they were stripey and kind of bulky. I have photos of myself wearing those in with a singlet top. And my singlet top tucked in! So I've got these bulky shorts that were past my knees and very baggy with a singlet top tucked in neatly.

It's the sort of thing, when I see these photos, it's just laughter all around. If my girlfriend Ally had met me back then, I'd have had no chance. But at the time I had no doubt that I looked ok.

What's the most important thing your dad taught you?

Dad never really gave me any fashion tips; just to try and dress reasonably smart. But again, he was always on about good manners and opening the door for your mother. Even this morning walking to work, I carried my partner's bags for her. Yesterday she was heading home from the market and I knew she had her arms full, so I met her half way, so I could carry all the things.

I think it's great to keep chivalry alive. It's not dead, but in today's society, it's definitely being let go of as the norm.

What style advice would you give to young guys?

I think it's probably all those things that you talk about; try to buy things that you love.

One thing I try to do is not to regret any decisions and I'm happy to always spend a little extra to get something that is high quality. And keep it simple.

Why keep it simple?

That way you just can't get it wrong. I just want to keep things simple and stylish and it's how I feel most comfortable and most relaxed.

What is your favorite piece?

My tailored jacket. It was a gift from Ally. She went to Hong Kong on business and, being a fashion designer, she measured me up and took the measurements to a tailor. It's a beautiful material and it was a gift made with love. It's just gorgeous. I don't know if it's the right term, but it's a 'signature piece' in my wardrobe.

What's on your wish list?
I guess a fabulous classic leather jacket would be nice. Maybe another blazer. A bit more casual perhaps. Keeping it simple, I don't really want too many clothes. I just don't need lots of shoes or shirts or jackets—I'm all about minimal. I live in my Yoga kit most of the time, as it's my everyday work uniform.

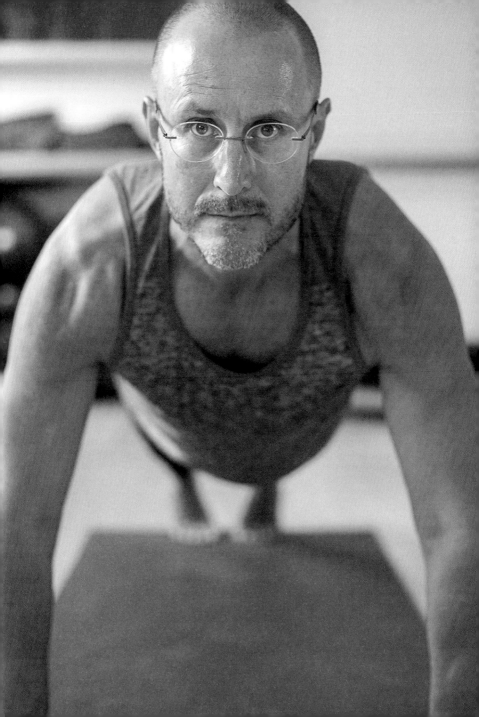

Thank you to Ali Cotton, Rick Tilelli, Daniel Rowntree, Stephen Foyle, Richard Shemesian, Robert Ian Bonnick, Ian MacDougall, Glenn Redman, Glen Carlson, Travis Wade, Robert Carroll, Gary Lack, Layla Saleeba, Alicia Albiston, Mark Ferguson, Simone Landes, Renee Stekel, Alex Zabotto Bentley, Dion Horstmans, Peter Hill, Luc Wiesman, Andrew Hampson, Brent Wilson, Luca Bronzino and Will Nhongo.

Peace and love JL

PHOTO CREDITS

Special thanks to Samantha Mackie for the wonderful work she did photographing the images for this book. Samantha Mackie Photography, www.samanthamackie.com

Cover image: Tom Antcliff, Photographer www.tomantcliff.com

A special thanks to the individuals and companies who gave their time during the production of this book.

Neighbourhood, neighbourhoodbondi.com.au
Harrolds, harrolds.com.au
Detail for Men, detailformen.com
Perfect Vision, perfectvisionoptical.com
Strand Hatters, strandhatters.com.au
Body Mind Life, bodymindlife.com
Belance, belance.com.au
Wil Valor, wilvalor.com.au
Neuw, neuwdenim.com
MJ Bale, mjbale.com.au
AS Colour, ascolour.com.au
G&L Handmade, gandlshoes.com
Declic, declic.com.au

First published in 2015 by New Holland Publishers Pty Ltd
London · Sydney · Auckland

The Chandlery Unit 009 50 Westminster Bridge Road London SE1 7QY
United Kingdom
1/66 Gibbes Street Chatswood NSW 2067 Australia
5/39 Woodside Ave Northcote, Auckland 0627 New Zealand

Copyright © 2015 New Holland Publishers Pty Ltd
Copyright © 2015 in text: Jeff Lack
Copyright © 2015 in images: See photo credits.

All rights reserved. No part of this publication may be reproduced,
stored in a retrieval system or transmitted, in any form or by any means,
electronic, mechanical, photocopying, recording or otherwise, without the
prior written permission of the publishers and copyright holders.

A record of this book is held at the British Library and the National
Library of Australia.

ISBN: 9781742577715

Managing Director: Fiona Schultz
Publisher: Diane Ward
Project Editor: Susie Stevens
Designer: Andrew Quinlan
Production Director: Olga Dementiev
Printer: Toppan Leefung Printing Limited
10 9 8 7 6 5 4 3 2 1

Keep up with New Holland Publishers on Facebook
www.facebook.com/NewHollandPublishers

US: $19.99
UK: £16.99